STAYING YOUNG WITH
INTERVAL TRAINING

Dr. Joseph Tieri

The Revolutionary HIIT Approach to Getting Fit, Living Healthy and Keeping Muscles Young

T0058131

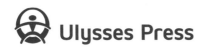

Published in the United States by:
Ulysses Press
P.O. Box 3440
Berkeley, CA 94703
www.ulyssespress.com

ISBN13: 978-1-61243-780-4
Library of Congress Control Number 2018930780

Printed in the United States by Kingery Printing Company, United Graphics Division

10 9 8 7 6 5 4 3 2 1

Acquisitions editor: Casie Vogel
Managing editor: Claire Chun
Editors: Shayna Keyles, Lily Chou
Proofreader: Renee Rutledge
Indexer: Sayre Van Young
Front cover design: Chris Cote
Cover artwork: © wavebreakmedia/shutterstock.com
Interior design and layout: what!design @ whatweb.com
Models: Andrew Hillman, Kym Sterner

Distributed by Publishers Group West

Please note: This book has been written and published strictly for informational purposes, and in no way should be used as a substitute for consultation with health care professionals. You should not consider educational material herein to be the practice of medicine or to replace consultation with a physician or other medical practitioner. The author and publisher are providing you with information in this work so that you can have the knowledge and can choose, at your own risk, to act on that knowledge. The author and publisher also urge all readers to be aware of their health status and to consult health care professionals before beginning any health program.

For my loving wife Janice and my two precious daughters Alexis and Madison

CONTENTS

INTRODUCTION

If you're reading this book, you're obviously interested in getting into better physical shape. And you likely fall into one of three categories:

1. You're a real fitness buff, and you're always looking for the latest, greatest thing for your workouts.

2. You're not that passionate about exercise just for exercise's sake—you dread the idea of long workouts on treadmills and stationary bikes—but you understand the importance of fitness and are looking for the best, most enjoyable way to get into better shape.

3. You don't want to have anything to do with exercise. You neither enjoy it nor think you have time for it. However, you've either been told, or deep-down know, that you should do it for your health.

Well, I have some great news for you. The approach to fitness laid out in this book will satisfy you no matter which group you fall into. Let me introduce you to a category of exercise known as High-Intensity Interval Training (HIIT). This relatively new and exciting form of exercise can:

1. Maximize the fitness benefits for exercise junkies.

2. Make exercising much more varied and enjoyable for those who need it to be fun.

3. Give impressive health results, in a minimal amount of time, for those who feel about exercise the way a three-year-old feels about eating vegetables.

Sound too good to be true? That's what I thought before I considered HIIT. As you'll discover in the pages that follow, there's some very exciting new research that touts the benefits of HIIT. It not only compares the benefits of HIIT to being a couch potato, but also to more common and popular forms of exercise like walking, jogging, or cycling—referred to as Moderate Intensity Continuous Training (MICT) in science jargon.

In almost every category, the fitness benefits of HIIT over MICT are significant and obvious. In a few other cases, you can reap the same or similar health benefits in *much* less time using HIIT. Whether you're interested in better health, fitness, strength, or weight loss, you'll succeed with HIIT not by exercising more but by exercising smarter. Say goodbye to 30-minute jogs, 45-minute bike rides, and hour-long walks—save them for Sundays with the grandkids!

How to Use This Book

This one is simple: I highly recommend that you just keep reading this book straight through. The chapters are easy to read and full of very important information to give you the best experience possible. Before going forward, however, please be aware that, as with all exercise programs, HIIT can challenge your body and is not without risk. As a physician, I strongly recommend that, before you ramp up your exercise activity, you consult your own doctor. Depending on your medical condition and history, you may need to be cleared before engaging in vigorous exercise or directly supervised during training.

Chapter One, "Staying Young with HIIT," is in some ways the soul of the book because it reveals all the amazing benefits you can expect from HIIT. For most people, it will be the source of motivation and their reason *why*—the reason that they strap their sneakers on a couple of times a week.

Chapter Two, "Getting Started the Right Way," is perhaps the most important chapter in the book. To be successful with your workouts and avoid injury, it's very important that your body be prepared. In my first book, *End Everyday Pain for 50+: A 10-Minute-a-Day Program of Stretching, Strengthening, and Movement to Break the Grip of Pain*, I recommended that people prepare their body by stretching and doing other movement exercises before engaging in fitness. It's no different here. In fact, since these exercises are more intense than some people are accustomed to, it may even be more important. This chapter includes some valuable information on how to proceed if you have pain or physical limitations, information on nutrition and supplementation, methods for assessing your fitness level, and recommendations on goal-setting for your new fitness journey. This will help get you started—and keep you going—the right way.

Chapter Three, "Dynamic Warm-Up," provides information on the importance of dynamic warm-up stretches. Proper warming up is essential to get the most out of your exercise experience. These warm-ups serve to further prepare and condition your body for the workouts and help you avoid injury.

Chapter Four, "HIIT Routines," begins with information on optional exercise gear you can acquire to enhance your workout experience. It also gives you specific HIIT routines, from beginner to more advanced, and includes a specialty routine specifically for postural improvement.

Chapter Five, "The HIIT Exercises," describes more than 40 step-by-step high-intensity interval exercises organized into upper-body, lower-body, core, and aerobic (cardio) exercises.

The Appendix details a number of foam roller exercises used for cooling down, as well as static stretches that help get your body more limber and accepting. The stretches also release tension and improve alignment, which often assist in decreasing or eliminating chronic pain and improving one's level of function and enjoyment of life.

Mental Blocks

Unless you're one of the lucky few who fall into the first category listed on page 7 (the real fitness buff), you'll likely need some help with motivation. No matter how important something may be to your health and well-being—and, as you'll find out in the next chapter, there are amazing, scientifically proven benefits of HIIT in just about every health category—there are always mental blocks preventing you from doing it. The most common barriers to exercise are:

1. Not understanding why you need to exercise

2. Thinking you don't have enough time to exercise

3. Seeing exercise as all work and no play

4. Not having access to enjoyable ways to exercise

The first key to making changes, to getting started with any valuable endeavor, is to have a big enough *why*. Hopefully, after reading through the next chapter, you'll have a clear understanding of the powerful benefits of HIIT and agree that it's essential to optimal health. Understanding your personal *why*, however, is so important that we'll cover it in more detail when we discuss goal-setting in Chapter Two.

Thinking you don't have enough time for exercise is also a major hurdle to beginning and maintaining an exercise routine. Studies have demonstrated that many people withdraw from exercise programs, citing lack of time as the main reason. (Of course, a lack of time may just be a cover for a lack of interest, in which case it goes back to the first barrier of not understanding why you need to exercise.) Thankfully, because HIIT can deliver all those amazing physical and mental benefits in a fraction of the time it takes for more traditional moderate-pace exercise—as little as 10 minutes two or three times a week—you'll discover that it can easily fit into your schedule.

So, what about the third and fourth barriers? Is HIIT more fun than traditional exercise, and more readily accessible? Well, that last one is easy. As this book will show you, having the ability to do these exercise routines in your basement, den, exercise room, or office makes them very accessible.

As far as the fun factor goes, while it would be misleading to say that HIIT isn't work (because it is), several studies have shown HIIT to be more enjoyable to exercise newcomers than regular MICT exercise is. In one study, 92 percent of participants found HIIT to be more enjoyable than MICT because it takes less time and the activities vary.[1]

This last point is important. Boredom has always been one of the biggest obstacles to continued exercise. Personally, I've always found beginning a 30- to 45-minute MICT routine to be mentally challenging. Even at 10 minutes in, the thought of the rest of the workout can be difficult to swallow. I've suffered through long, mundane treadmill workouts, trying to reduce the boredom by watching TV. By keeping the HIIT intervals short, changing up the routines, and constantly adding new elements to a workout, exercise can stay interesting and, yes, fun. That also explains why studies have frequently demonstrated that participants in HIIT workouts perceive them to be less intense (using a self-reporting scale called Rate of Perceived Exertion, or RPE) than MICT.

Why HIIT?

I wrote my first book, *End Everyday Pain for 50+*, to warn about the common experience of middle-aged people suffering from a seemingly sudden breakdown of their musculoskeletal system as they aged. In reality, there's nothing sudden about it. Without adopting preventive measures—like stretching and strengthening—the forgiving nature of youth slowly segues into the alternating and recurrent neck, shoulder, back, hip, and knee pain of middle and older age. Armed with the information from that book, plus 10 minutes a day of action, people discovered that they could reduce or eliminate the chronic pain and problems from these common trouble spots.

This time, I've written a book to educate people about a different set of problems that might come their way (the possibility of premature heart disease, strokes, diabetes, and dementia) if they don't begin a preventive fitness routine. And don't be fooled into thinking that it's good enough to just be a very active person or, as my patients say, to "never sit down," or to "go up and down the stairs all day long." It's true that by being active, it takes more time for you to get weaker and less fit. But unless you challenge your body by asking it to do something it can't already do, it won't get any stronger or fitter. The body's smart that way. It won't put any extra resources into building itself up if it can already do what's asked of it. It's always looking to conserve energy.

Fortunately, your body's challenge is here: HIIT, the most powerful and efficient health and fitness program there is. And yes, you'll be tested. You must be. And by accepting that physical challenge, you'll also reap all the mental benefits that go with it. So, congratulations on buying this book and taking the first step toward being in the best possible shape you can be so that you can enjoy the healthy life you deserve.

Now let's take a closer look at some of the science to discover why HIIT has become so popular over the last few years.

CHAPTER ONE

STAYING YOUNG WITH HIIT

We know that aging occurs at the cellular level. However, more and more studies are revealing that exercise creates positive changes at the cellular and genetic level, affecting the very building blocks of the body. A 2017 study reported in *Preventive Medicine* found that the more exercise people got, the less aging their cells experienced.[2] People who exercised at least 30 to 40 minutes a day, five days a week had biological aging markers *nine years younger* than those who didn't exercise at all. Imagine turning 65 years old and removing 9 candles from your birthday cake and, voila, you're 56! As evidenced by their cells, those who exercise not only have a better chance of living longer, they also develop fewer chronic diseases.[3] Who wouldn't like to live longer and healthier as well?

And wouldn't it be nice if you could get the same health and longevity results, *or better*, in a fraction of the time? Well, the good news is that with HIIT, you can. It just well might be the fountain of youth.

But before we delve into the exciting new research about the time-saving health and fitness benefits of HIIT, let's talk more about what HIIT actually is.

What Is High-Intensity Interval Training?

High-intensity interval training, or **HIIT**, is not a type of exercise or a set routine. At its essence, HIIT is a way of exercising characterized by variety. The most important element of variety in HIIT is pacing, or the level of exertion invested. Short intervals of higher-intensity exercise are alternated with intervals of lower-intensity effort, also known as rest, or recovery, periods.

So instead of an exercise routine consisting of a steady, moderate-pace activity like walking, cycling on flat roads, or lifting weights on a circuit at a gym, a high-intensity routine might consist of a warm-up period followed by short bouts of jogging, fast running, hard cycling, or short sets of lifting light weights rapidly, followed by recovery periods of walking, slower jogging, slower pedaling, or just resting between weightlifting sets.

While you can achieve this variety by alternating the intensity levels of a single activity, as in the previous examples, a popular form of HIIT also varies the types of exercise in each workout. A workout can include exercises of a similar type, like all cardio or all strength-training, or it can include both types of exercises within a single session. Not only can varying the type of exercise make it more interesting and fun, but it also offers a more challenging and complete workout for the body.

The level of exertion typically achieved in the more commonly practiced MICT exercises equates to about 60 percent of your maximal heart rate, defined as the maximum beats per minute (bpm) achieved without overexerting yourself. In contrast, during the high-intensity portion of an HIIT workout, the goal is to get your heart rate up to at least 80 percent of your maximal heart rate (approaching 90+ percent for very fit people), and have it drop down to approximately 40 percent of maximal heart rate during the rest, or recovery, period. Realize that these are relative measures, meaning the intensity required to really get your heart pumping will be different for a fit 50-year-old versus an out-of-shape 65-year-old.

Though more precise ways of calculating maximal heart rate exist, for most people, the standard way is still fine:

MAXIMAL HEART RATE = 220 – YOUR AGE

Jane is 60 years old. Her maximal heart rate is 220 - 60 = 160. 160 represents the maximum heart rate she should ever achieve while exercising. During the brief high-intensity portion of Jane's HIIT workout, the goal is to get her heart rate to 80 percent of her maximum, or 128 bpm. During the rest or recovery intervals, it could drop back down to 96 bpm, which is 60 percent of her maximal rate.

Since not everyone monitors their pulse while exercising, here's a general rule to gauge how hard your heart is working. During MICT exercise, you should be able to carry on a conversation with your exercise partner with only periodic breaks to take a deep breath. In contrast, during the high-intensity portion of a HIIT exercise, having a conversation with someone would be very difficult. The best you'd be able to do is get a couple of words out between gasps of air. If you can carry on a normal conversation, you aren't exercising hard enough.

Here's another way to gauge your level of exertion during the high-intensity portion of interval training: If 10/10 represents running for your life, you want to feel that you're exercising at a level 8/10 (or 9/10, as you get fitter). You should be panting and sweating!

Though short, it's these intervals of high-intensity exertion that deliver most of the incredible benefits that science is discovering about HIIT.

How Short Can You Go?

Just how short are high-intensity intervals? Some of the earliest research was based on four 4-minute workouts that consisted of eight 20-second high-intensity exercise intervals, each interspersed with 10-second intervals of rest. Later studies have experimented with different interval lengths, most fitting within a 20-minute total time commitment and included warm-up and cool-down periods.

More recently, the term *reduced-exertion* high-intensity interval training (REHIIT) has been introduced. Several studies have shown significant fitness and cardiovascular benefits with *one minute or less* of high-intensity exercise! One such study, published in 2017, compared the impact of three 10-minute REHIIT exercise sessions per week to five 30-minute sessions of moderate-intensity walking for eight weeks. Each 10-minute workout consisted of just two "all-out" 10- to 20-second sprints. The results demonstrated a significantly larger aerobic effect in the REHIIT group, even with only one-fifth of the time spent exercising.[4]

Additionally, studies have also found significantly improved metabolic, cardiovascular, and fitness benefits in as little as six HIIT sessions performed over two weeks. A 2010 study published in *Metabolism* showed beneficial changes to insulin sensitivity, maximal oxygen uptake, systolic blood pressure, and waist and hip circumference in overweight sedentary men.[5] Imagine, measurable beneficial changes to health in just two weeks!

This is amazing new science and very exciting stuff. Exercise for health and fitness used to be about time invested, but now it's more about the intensity level. The time needed for an effective workout keeps shrinking.

HIIT, Muscle & Cellular Health

Research suggests that HIIT may undo some of the aging process. A Mayo Clinic study compared participants aged 64 to 80 to those aged 18 to 30. Subjects exercised three times a week for 12 weeks in one of three ways: HIIT exercise, vigorous upper- and lower-body weight training, and a combination of moderate-pace cycling and light weight training (MICT). The study found that "HIIT robustly improved cardio-respiratory fitness, insulin sensitivity, mitochondrial respiration, and fat-free mass in both age groups."[6]

The researchers also biopsied the muscle cells of the participants. According to some estimates, these muscles get steadily weaker after our mid-40s and don't regenerate easily. Amazingly, it was discovered that, by far, the largest number of gene changes occurred in the 64- to 80-year-old age group that participated in HIIT exercise. "HIIT robustly increased gene expression, particularly in older adults…HIIT also had robust increases in transcriptional and translational regulation of muscle growth and mitochondrial pathways."[7]

Exercise-Induced Gene Transformation

	AGE 18 TO 30	AGE 64 TO 80
HIIT	274	396
WEIGHT TRAINING	74	33
MICT	170	19

These results mean that the researchers discovered that the older people who participated in HIIT had cells with a significantly improved ability to regulate and control their own activity, which in turn resulted in improved cellular health. In addition, the mitochondria (the energy producers of the cell), which normally diminish as we get older, grew healthier and increased in numbers by almost 70 percent.

The HIIT group experienced the greatest overall health and fitness gains, including increased muscle strength and the strongest gains in endurance. In addition, the 64- to 80-year-old HIIT participants had, by far, the most dramatic changes in cellular health. This prompted the author of a study review article, quoting one of the principles of the study, to conclude, "It seems as if the decline in the cellular health of muscles associated with aging was 'corrected' with exercise, especially if [the exercise] was intense."[8]

Telomere Length

A telomere is the cap at the end of a chromosome that protects it from damage. Every time a cell divides, the telomeres shorten, exposing the cell to damage. Telomerase is an enzyme that attempts to replenish the shortening telomere and protect the cell from death. HIIT has a positive impact on telomerase, too: A 2014 study reported in the *International Journal of Analytical, Pharmaceutical and Biomedical Sciences* examined the effects of HIIT exercise on young sedentary women. The women exercised three times per week for eight weeks. In addition to significant decreases in body fat, body mass index, and weight, the women who participated in HIIT saw a significant increase in telomerase activity, and consequently in telomere length.[9]

Now that you've suffered through a crash course in genetics, you can see that the benefits of HIIT go to the very depths of your being. They reverse some age-related decline, protect your

DNA, and improve the health and longevity of your cells—all the while preventing disease and prolonging your life. If that's not the fountain of youth, I don't know what is!

HIIT & Disease Prevention

Over the last 20 years of my medical practice, I've treated thousands of adults who aged from their mid-50s into their 60s and 70s. Many were health conscious and physically active; others were not. Without a doubt, those that didn't exercise regularly declined physically and mentally at a much faster rate.

And, unfortunately, modern medicine won't necessarily come to the rescue when things fall apart later in life. Though great strides have been made and many lifesaving techniques exist, the quality of life with diabetes, or after suffering a heart attack or getting a joint replacement, isn't always rosy. The side effects of medication often result in a poorer quality of life. Muscle pain and fatigue are common side effects, and some of my patients have had to give up hobbies they love, like gardening and woodworking, because they're on blood thinners and fear cutting themselves. Studies also show that a significant number of people still have pain and are unhappy with their replaced joints following surgery.

Don't get to the point where you wish you had taken better care of yourself. You must be proactive and take personal ownership of your health. It's easy to do, and ultimately, very physically and mentally rewarding.

Now, let's talk more about some of the specific medical and fitness benefits of HIIT.

Cardiovascular Health

Nowhere are the benefits of HIIT more notable than on the healthy functioning of the heart. According to the American Heart Association, approximately one of every three deaths in the US is caused by cardiovascular disease. That's nearly 2,200 deaths a day, or about one death every 40 seconds. The average age for a first heart attack is 65 for males and 72 for females. Unfortunately, these statistics are projected to get worse in the coming years.

Fortunately, by altering your lifestyle, you can drastically reduce the odds of suffering from cardiovascular disease. There's likely nothing that will have more of an impact on the healthy functioning of the cardiovascular system than exercise because of its impacts on resting heart rate, insulin sensitivity, blood pressure, cholesterol, and body fat.

In a 2005 study published in the *Journal of Applied Physiology*, previously sedentary men were randomly placed into HIIT or MICT exercise groups for a total of 24 weeks. At the end of that time, tests revealed that in addition to a greater improvement in participants' fitness levels, only the HIIT group achieved significant improvement in total cholesterol, LDL cholesterol, and non-

HDL cholesterol. The changes in cholesterol were deemed sufficient to decrease coronary heart disease (CHD) incidence by 54 percent, prompting the authors to conclude that "…high-intensity exercise should be performed if the goal of training is to maximize cardiorespiratory fitness. The present study also suggests that changes in CHD risk factors are influenced by exercise intensity."[10]

As reported in a 2017 *British Journal of Sports Medicine*, a systematic review of 65 studies demonstrated that short-term HIIT, defined as less than 12 weeks of exercise, significantly improves diastolic blood pressure and fasting blood sugar levels in overweight populations. Meanwhile, long-term HIIT, defined as more than 12 weeks of exercise, significantly improved resting heart rate, as well as systolic and diastolic blood pressure, in overweight populations.[11]

Additionally, it has been established that poor cardiorespiratory fitness is the result of people's lifestyle choices, resulting in coronary artery disease, heart failure, hypertension, metabolic syndrome, and obesity. The conclusion of a 2014 review and analysis of data from 10 qualifying studies was: "HIIT significantly increases cardiorespiratory fitness by almost double that of MICT in patients with lifestyle-induced chronic diseases."[12]

Whether you'd like to decrease your heart disease incidence by 54 percent, improve your blood pressure and blood sugar levels in less than 12 weeks, or almost double your fitness benefit in half the time, HIIT is the vehicle. Impressive, I'd say!

Cardiovascular Risk?

While it's clear that HIIT provides significant benefits to your cardiovascular system, it's natural to wonder if an exercise that's more intense might be too risky to your heart. And while it's true that exercising in the upper limits of your maximal heart rate will cause the heart to work harder, the science seems to say it's as safe as engaging in moderate forms of exercise, and safer than not exercising at all.

A 2012 study reported in the journal *Circulation* examined the risk of cardiovascular events during high-intensity interval exercise versus moderate-intensity exercise among almost 5,000 patients with coronary artery disease who were staying in cardiac rehabilitation centers. They concluded that "…the risk of a cardiovascular event is low after both high-intensity exercise and moderate-intensity exercise…Considering the significant cardiovascular adaptations associated with high-intensity exercise, such exercise should be considered among the patients with coronary heart disease."[13]

Keep in mind that the above study took place in a cardiac rehab setting, so make sure that, if you have a history of cardiovascular disease or high blood pressure, you get clearance from your cardiologist since you'll likely be exercising in an unsupervised setting.

It's also vital for your heart health that you not jump into any exercise program too fast. As we'll discuss more in Chapter Two, it's important that you begin slowly and build up to a comfortable level of exercise. Too much of any type of exercise (also known as overtraining) can have diminishing, and even negative, returns.

It's nice to report that while the program is more intense, people have generally found HIIT to be well-tolerated. The 2005 study from the *Journal of Applied Physiology*, referenced on page 15, had this to say: "…the present study is in agreement with those of others who found no difference in injury or dropout rates between moderate- and high-intensity exercise groups."[14]

Brain Health & Alzheimer's

A significant number of adults over age 60 already have dementia and, by age 65, 1 in 10 people are afflicted with Alzheimer's disease, a form of dementia that is the fifth leading cause of death among seniors.[15] Toward the end of life, 1 in 3 seniors is affected. A new case of Alzheimer's is detected every 66 seconds.

The importance of preventing or slowing down cognitive decline and the development of Alzheimer's disease and other forms of dementia cannot be overstated. The toll it takes on patients and families alike can be significant. Symptoms of this devastating disease include impairment in memory, behavior, and mood, and the inability to handle complex tasks like managing money and driving.

While not that long ago, there was no clear evidence about the effects of lifestyle on the onset of dementia—in fact, the Alzheimer's Association website still claims it's the only top ten cause of death that cannot be prevented, cured, or even slowed—I'm happy to report that that may be changing. According to *Prevention* magazine, citing a study published in the *American Journal of Physiology*, while not specifically about interval training, a study conducted at the University of Texas Southwestern Medical Center followed almost 20,000 people over the course of 38 years, evaluating their midlife fitness levels and the later-life development of all-cause dementia (Alzheimer's disease, as well as other types of dementia). The study concluded that "higher midlife fitness levels seem to be associated with lower hazards of developing all-cause dementia later in life."[16]

Another important study, this one conducted at the University of Illinois, followed 59 inactive individuals between the ages of 60 and 79. Over a six-month period, half of them were enrolled into an aerobic training regimen, and the other half participated in a toning and stretching program. Researchers took 3D MRIs of the regions of the brain associated with age-related decline both before and after the exercise intervals. The results found significant volume increases in both gray and white matter regions of the brain only for those who participated in the aerobic training.

The authors concluded that "…cardiovascular fitness is associated with the sparing of brain tissue in aging humans…these results suggest a strong biological basis for the role of aerobic fitness in maintaining and enhancing central nervous system health and cognitive functioning in older adults."[17]

The take-home message of these studies is that, in addition to all the other known health benefits of exercise, it also positively affects the brain and its ability to function. And while the University of Texas study showed the importance of getting fit in midlife, which positively affected brain functioning years later, the University of Illinois study noted that positive changes are possible in just six months for a group of older individuals.

Although these studies weren't specifically about HIIT, there's no reason to think that you can't get similar results—in much less time—with HIIT!

Stroke Prevention

A stroke is the sudden death of brain cells, most commonly from a blockage of an artery that delivers blood and oxygen to the cells. Complications include loss of speech, weakness, and paralysis, making strokes one of the leading causes of serious long-term disability. According to the American Heart Association, someone in the US suffers from a stroke approximately every 40 seconds, and someone dies from a stroke every four minutes. While this represents a serious problem, most strokes are fortunately preventable with lifestyle changes.

According to a study published in the *American Journal of Physiology*, HIIT performed twice a week for 12 weeks positively influenced estrogen levels and markers associated with the hardening of the arteries in post-menopausal women, reducing their risk of stroke by 40 percent.[18] Additionally, a 2015 Australian study reviewed and analyzed the data of seven randomized trials comparing HIIT and MICT. The study focused on the effects of the exercises on vascular function, noting that vascular dysfunction significantly increases the chance of cardiovascular events, including stroke. On average, participants in the studies engaged in HIIT three times per week for 12 to 16 weeks. Among the many positive effects reported for HIIT was that it was more effective at improving brachial artery vascular function than MICT. Authors concluded that it "…is a powerful form of exercise to enhance vascular function."[19]

Diabetes Prevention

Diabetes dramatically increases the risk of heart attacks and strokes, as well as disabling nerve, kidney, and eye damage. Approximately 30 million Americans are afflicted with this serious medical condition, and another 8 million are likely afflicted but undiagnosed. What's perhaps more alarming is that the Centers for Disease Control and Prevention (CDC) reports that another 86 million American adults—more than one in three—are estimated to have prediabetes, a condition characterized by higher-than-normal blood sugar levels, but not yet high enough to be classified as type 2 diabetes. Without intervention, approximately 15 to 30 percent of those adults will have the disease within five years.

While these statistics are worrying, and immediate action is certainly needed to prevent and treat this debilitating condition, the good news is that it's well known that exercise is one of the most effective means to improve the regulation of blood sugar. And HIIT is proving to be particularly effective. In a study conducted in Denmark, a group of non-active adults in their 50s, some with type 2 diabetes and some without, participated in HIIT exercises three times a week for eight weeks. The results of the study were impressive. Both the non-diabetic and diabetic participants benefited from significant abdominal fat loss. Diabetic participants enjoyed significant improvements in blood sugar and insulin categories, as well as improved pancreatic b-cell function, prompting the authors to conclude: "The study provides evidence for the health benefits of eight weeks of HIIT in type 2 diabetics."[20] Similarly, as reported in a 2017 *British Journal of Sports Medicine* study, short-term HIIT—defined as less than 12 weeks of exercise—significantly improves fasting sugar levels in overweight populations.[21]

Whether you're one of the 38 million Americans with diabetes, diagnosed or not, or one of the one in three Americans in a prediabetic state, the great news is that just eight weeks of exercise can significantly improve how your body processes sugar. When combined with diet, appropriate exercise can reduce or prevent this deadly disease.

Weight Loss

Losing excess weight bridges the gap between medical benefits and fitness gains. If you're overweight, losing even as little as 5 percent of that weight can reduce your risk of acquiring certain diseases and cancers due to improvements in any one of several areas, like blood pressure, cholesterol, and insulin sensitivity. In the fitness category, weight loss can decrease the load on your muscles and joints, and improve your sleep, energy level, and mood.

The studies are clear: HIIT is the best way to lose weight. Not only does it appear that you burn more fat when your exercise intensity is higher, but in some cases, moderate-pace exercise may not even lead to any of the fat loss observed in HIIT. This may not come as a surprise to you, since many people have difficulty losing weight even when engaging in typical forms of aerobic exercise.

Take the following two studies as examples. A 2016 study compared the effects of 20 minutes of HIIT compared to 40 minutes of MICT performed twice a week for 16 weeks in postmenopausal women with type 2 diabetes. The results showed that overall fat mass decreased and that significant loss of abdominal and visceral fat mass—also known as central obesity, the type most commonly associated with disease—was observed only with HIIT.[22]

In another study, this one from 2008, 45 young women participated in a 15-week cycling exercise program. The women participating in the HIIT exercise did three 20-minute sessions per week, and the women enrolled in the steady-state exercise did three 40-minute session per week. While both exercise groups got significantly fitter, only the HIIT group had a significant reduction in total body mass, fat mass, and leg and trunk fat.[23]

Even in those studies that discover similarities in weight-loss measures between HIIT and MICT, HIIT participants achieve their results in much less time. One such 2017 study, reported in *Obesity Review*, found that both high-intensity and moderate-intensity exercise produced significant reductions in whole-body fat mass and waist circumference. They concluded that "HIIT and MICT show similar effectiveness across all body composition measures, suggesting that HIIT may be a time-efficient component of weight-management programs."[24]

The bottom line: HIIT results in equal to greater weight loss and body reshaping—in half the time!

HIIT & Fitness

The fitness benefits of HIIT have been known for many years, mainly in the circles of elite athletes training at the highest levels. Even professional athletes who compete in moderate-paced sports—like distance runners and cyclists—discovered that they could perform better in their sport by adding high-intensity interval training to their workouts.

HIIT has more recently filtered down into the realms of amateur athletes and fitness buffs, mainly through programs offered at gyms and other facilities. These workout programs are sometimes referred to as Tabata, named after Izumi Tabata, the Japanese speed-skating coach and professor who co-authored a 1996 study extolling the fitness benefits of HIIT. The original protocol utilized cycling ergometers. After a 5-minute warm-up, the regimen consisted of eight 20-second intervals of high-intensity pedaling broken up with 10-second rest periods—4 minutes total—followed by a 2-minute cool-down period.

While Izumi Tabata's study proved the value of HIIT with elite athletes, numerous studies since then have utilized non-athletes to confirm the fitness benefits. One such study, published in the *Journal of Applied Physiology*, followed previously sedentary men, who were randomly placed into either MICT or HIIT exercise groups, for 24 weeks. After the study, the authors determined that HIIT is more effective than MICT in increasing VO2 max.[25] (Also known as maximal oxygen uptake, VO2 max is a measure of the maximum rate of oxygen consumption during incremental exercise, and is a reliable marker for aerobic physical fitness level.) Other studies have also demonstrated that even short-term HIIT, defined as less than 12 weeks of exercise, significantly improved VO2 max. Long-term HIIT—participation in HIIT for longer than 12 weeks—significantly improved waist circumference, percentage of body fat, and VO2 max in overweight populations.[26]

Of course, the fitness benefits of exercise are inseparable from the health benefits. The more fit you are, the healthier you are. Numerous studies have demonstrated that a high level of fitness is associated with a lower rate of death from any cause. Whether your goal is to be fitter or healthier, HIIT is a great way to get there.

Strengthening

By some estimates, our muscles get at least 5 percent weaker every decade starting in our 40s, accelerating to 15 percent per decade once we reach our 60s, assuming we don't intervene. And while some weakness is a normal result of aging, many problems for older people are due to neglect. That's why taking steps to maintain, and then build, strength become important objectives for people over 50.

Because of muscle weakness, many of my older patients begin to struggle with seemingly simple everyday tasks, like climbing stairs and getting up out of chairs. Balance issues and falls can also result, leading to hip fractures and other life-threatening injuries. The fear of falling affects confidence and the ability to engage fully in life. Perhaps most frustrating to many older people is the need to abandon long-loved hobbies, like gardening and golf, due to the physical limitations that a weaker body creates.

The good news is that the HIIT strengthening routines included in this book can help you avoid that fate. Also called resistance exercises, or calisthenics, they use your own body weight (although you may progress to using light weights eventually) to improve muscle strength— even in very elderly adults. They create the strong muscles and tendons that protect your joints, and they stress your bones, which prompts them to absorb minerals to get stronger and helps prevent osteoporosis and compression fractures of the spine.

The strengthening exercises included in this book target the upper body, the lower body, and the core. They're *compound* exercises, which are very efficient at strengthening many different muscles and joints at once. Performed one to three times per week, these exercises can reduce pain from muscles and joints, decrease frailty, and reduce the risk of falls. The strength-training exercises can also increase confidence, reduce stress and anxiety, improve mood, and keep you active and engaged long into your twilight years. In addition, because they're done in a HIIT aerobic exercise format, they can also give you all the incredible medical health benefits we've talked about already.

Afterburn

Your body continues to burn calories after you've finished your workout, while you're resting on the couch. This is referred to as "afterburn," also known as Excess Post-Exercise Oxygen Consumption (EPOC). The demanding nature of HIIT creates a situation in which the body must continue to work to restore itself to its pre-exercise state once you've finished your workout. Many studies report that this continued burning of calories is more significant after high-intensity and resistance-type workouts, two components frequently found in HIIT programs.

What this means to you, of course, is a body that continues to lose weight after you've finished your workout, kind of like money in the bank earning interest while you sleep. As the authors of one study put it, "…the positive news is that any additional caloric expenditure following exercise can add up over time and may contribute to long-term weight management."[27]

The Time Is Now

Are you starting to see why you need to exercise? I hope so. Do you still think you don't have enough time for it? I hope not. If you're convinced that the quality of your health is at stake and you're ready to get started, then let's move on and learn how to exercise the right way.

CHAPTER TWO

GETTING STARTED THE RIGHT WAY

While some studies demonstrate that the benefits of HIIT can be even greater for an older age group, and though it's not necessarily riskier to your health than moderate forms of exercise are, there are some special considerations for those of us over 50.

Medical Clearance

No matter who you are, but especially if you're not well conditioned to exercise, you need to check in with your doctor and get medical clearance before embarking on any new physical fitness program. While this is true of all programs, it becomes especially important when the program includes high-intensity exercise levels. And don't let the shorter duration of these routines fool you: They're demanding, and you need to be sure you can handle them physically.

To avoid injury, it's important to receive a physical examination and clearance from your medical physician, particularly if you have a heart condition, are pregnant, have cancer or other serious medical illness, have osteoporosis, have had joint replacement surgery or other orthopedic problems, or have had other surgeries. Your doctor can also provide some baseline health-status measurements (see Fitness Assessment on page 29) so you can look back later and see how you've improved after starting your HIIT program.

Avoiding Injury

To prevent injury, it's important to prepare your body before engaging in exercise. I've treated thousands of middle- to older-age people over the course of my career, many of whom began an exercise program—walking, cycling, or working out at the gym—at the request of loved ones and cardiologists, only to be sidelined soon after by pain and injury. Most people don't fully realize that years of inactivity, compromising work and play habits, and inattention to their body creates tension and misalignment in their muscles and joints. Suddenly adding the repetitive motions inherent in most forms of exercise is a recipe for disaster.

Don't be in a hurry to start. Use the static stretches (see page 119) at least three to four times a week (although every day would be better) to begin the process of undoing years of accumulated strain, and adding more "space" to your body. A body with more space in it has an easier time handling the repetitive motion inherent in exercise. I also recommend you *slowly* add some dynamic warm-ups (see page 32) and foam roller exercises (see page 112) to further loosen and prepare your body. There's no exact formula for how long this will all take—it depends on your present condition—but a few weeks wouldn't be too much time for the average adult body.

Once prepared, it's also a good idea to do some moderate forms of light aerobic activity—walking, jogging, biking, or elliptical-type exercises—to get your cardiovascular system ready for the more intense bursts of exercises to come. The American Academy of Sports Medicine recommends that a baseline level of fitness be present before engaging in HIIT. They recommend 20 minutes or more of at least moderate-intensity aerobic exercise, at least a few times a week over several weeks, to prepare the muscles. I know you're probably eager to get started, but, ironically, think of this as a marathon and not a sprint (for now). You're going to want to be exercising for years to come. Patience and preparation will pay off!

Once you've begun the HIIT exercises, realize that while some generalized soreness is natural the day or two after a workout, pain that's more severe, that comes from a specific location, or that radiates may be more serious. Numbness, tingling, or burning sensations may also be signs that tension in the body is irritating a nerve. If any of these cases occur, you should take a few days off from exercise and, when the symptoms abate, begin again more slowly. If pain or problems worsen or persist, consult your medical or musculoskeletal expert.

How to Proceed If You Have Chronic Muscle or Joint Pain

Many of my middle- and older-age patients come to me for hands-on treatment because of chronic pain and problems in their muscles and joints, most commonly from the neck, shoulders, lower back, hips, or knees. These complaints are frequently the result of tension from poor posture—shoulders rounded, backs hunched over, feet and legs turned outward when walking—and the resultant weakness and misalignment.

You'll notice that I didn't blame the pain on radiologic findings like rotator cuff tears, herniated discs, arthritis, and meniscal tears. That's because, as my first book pointed out, these radiologic diagnoses are frequently artifacts of sorts and not the source of pain. Many studies bear this out, as a significant number of people who have no joint pain at all still receive these diagnoses when subjected to X-rays and MRIs.

What this means to you is that, if you have such diagnoses, you shouldn't assume they're the chief source of your pain and, as a result, either do nothing or feel obligated to seek a medical intervention like an injection or surgery. My advice is that, if possible, first attempt to treat the underlying problem using the same types of conservative care that studies prove can work: Address the postural imbalances, muscles tension, and weakness before resorting to more invasive medical approaches.

To that end, spend some time (a week or several, depending on the severity of the problem) doing the stretching, strengthening, and range-of-motion exercises for the problem area as recommended in my first book, *End Everyday Pain for 50+* (also see page 119 for some static stretches). To further realign your body and remove stress from problem areas, you may also consider getting treated by a good massage therapist, physical therapist, chiropractor, or osteopathic physician who does hands-on work.

In addition, follow the protocol listed in Avoiding Injury (page 24) by doing some dynamic warm-ups and foam roller exercises. Take your time with these; there's no hurry to begin the HIIT exercises in the book, and you don't want to have to stop before you've really started.

Lastly, choose exercises that don't cause you pain. If that nagging shoulder pain just won't go away, do some lower-body and core exercises. If, despite all your preparation, that hip just remains painful, do more upper-body exercises. This way you can still improve your overall fitness level while continuing to rehabilitate the injured and painful area. And because HIIT exercises can be done in much less time than traditional MICT exercises, they may be better tolerated by your body.

Start Low & Go Slow!

Not only the experience with my patients but also *my own* experience has taught me that it's very easy to overdo a new activity or exercise. Years ago, I did a set of dumbbell flys after not having done them in years. I didn't warm up, but also didn't think I was using overly heavy weights—I just figured I could pick up where I had left off. After all, I was only in my early 40s and didn't feel I had aged any. Well, I soon learned my lesson and had shoulder tendinitis, pain, and restricted motion for almost a year. Another time, I started running inclines on my new treadmill—having not run up hills in years—and spent the next nine months with hip pain from psoas tendinitis. And then there was the time I spent a couple of hours doing yardwork as soon as the spring thaw occurred--and I strained my wrist.

I think about these and other similar events whenever I pick up a new activity, or after taking a break from an old one—raking in the fall, shoveling in the winter, kicking a soccer ball in the spring—and really do go incredibly slowly in the beginning. It's how I keep myself out of trouble.

Use a Heart Rate Monitor

Monitoring your heart is a good way to ensure that you're not overworking it. Heart rate monitors come in all shapes and sizes, from ones you wear on your wrist to ones that strap around your chest. I have one that syncs up with my iPhone, which I put in a handlebar attachment on my bike. I like watching how my heart is responding during intense exercise, as well as during the recovery period. How quickly your heart returns to its baseline rate after a workout is one of the best markers of fitness level.

Nutrition

As you embark on the most advanced and effective fitness regimen to date, I recommend that you make some changes to your diet to support your journey. HIIT workouts, though short, demand a lot from your body. Putting the best fuel into your new high-octane engine, in the right proportions, will support your system and boost your results—whether you seek improved health and fitness or weight loss.

Your diet should be a balance of proteins, low-starch vegetables, complex carbohydrates, and good fats.

Quality Proteins. Try to select organic, grass-fed, free-range lean meats. They have no hormones or antibiotics, are naturally leaner, and can be higher in omega fats and other good nutrients. Protein can also be found in cheese, yogurt, eggs, soy, and fish.

Non-Starchy Vegetables. Non-starchy vegetables like spinach, cauliflower, and tomatoes contain fewer carbohydrates and calories compared to starchy vegetables like corn, peas, and potatoes.

Complex Carbohydrates. Carbohydrates are one of the body's main fuel sources and are vital in your diet as you engage in HIIT training. Simple carbohydrates should be avoided because they quickly break down into sugar once in the body. Instead, choose complex carbs like whole grains, beans, and apples, which take longer to break down and are higher in fiber.

Good Fats. Good sources of fat, such as avocados and nuts, help us lose weight, increase satiety, and increase metabolism. They're high in nutrients and free-radical-fighting antioxidants, and can protect against heart disease.

Some foods fall into more than one category, such as grass-fed beef and Greek yogurt, which are both good proteins and fats. To keep it simple, I recommend that you pick foods from this chart.

Foods to Eat

QUALITY PROTEINS	NON-STARCHY VEGETABLES	COMPLEX CARBOHYDRATES	GOOD FATS
✓ Beef	✓ Artichokes	✓ Apples	✓ Avocados
✓ Cheese	✓ Arugula	✓ Brown rice	✓ Butter
✓ Eggs	✓ Asparagus	✓ Chick peas	✓ Canola oil
✓ Greek yogurt	✓ Bok choy	✓ Grapefruit	✓ Coconut
✓ Pork	✓ Broccoli	✓ Kidney beans	✓ Dark chocolate
✓ Poultry (chicken, duck)	✓ Brussels sprouts	✓ Lentils	✓ Milk and heavy cream
✓ Salmon and other fish	✓ Cabbage	✓ Pears	✓ Nuts and nut butters, and seeds
✓ Soy products	✓ Carrots	✓ Prunes	✓ Olives
	✓ Cauliflower	✓ Quinoa	✓ Olive oil
	✓ Celery	✓ Split peas	
	✓ Cucumbers	✓ Strawberries	
	✓ Eggplant	✓ Tomatoes	
	✓ Escarole	✓ Whole grain breads (wheat, oat, multi-grain)	
	✓ Garlic	✓ Whole grain pasta	
	✓ Green beans	✓ Yogurt, low-fat	
	✓ Lettuce		
	✓ Mushrooms		
	✓ Onions		
	✓ Peppers		
	✓ Snow peas		
	✓ Spinach		
	✓ Summer squash		
	✓ Tomatoes		
	✓ Turnips		
	✓ Zucchini		

Avoid or limit these foods:

➡ Alcohol (limit to one or two drinks per day)

➡ Caffeine (limit to one to two cups per day, and pass on the sugar)

➡ Candy

➠ Pastries

➠ Processed foods and snacks

➠ Soda

➠ Starchy vegetables

➠ Trans fats (like margarine)

If your diet needs a lot of changes and clean-up, try to make a couple better choices each day, allowing your system to adjust. The urge to eat these foods will fade.

Depending on your current diet, you may benefit from increasing your intake of proteins (which are necessary for building and repairing muscle) and low-starch vegetables, adding some good fats, and reducing your non-complex carbohydrate intake. (But don't overdo it—you don't need to consume mass quantities of protein or to carbo-load for HIIT exercise.) This is a pretty standard weight-loss and fitness diet and, in some studies, it has been shown to reduce cholesterol levels and systemic inflammation. Always check with your physician before changing your diet, especially if you're pregnant, suffer from chronic medical problems, or take medication.

Here are some sample meals for any time:

➠ Eggs and cheese or lean breakfast meat on whole-grain toast

➠ Protein smoothie with berries, yogurt, and peanut or almond butter

➠ Salad greens with olive oil, vinegar, and shredded lunch meat

➠ Three-bean salad with avocado and tomato

➠ Caesar salad with grilled chicken, beef, or pork

➠ Grilled meat and roasted vegetables with brown rice or quinoa

Food & Your Workouts

Before, during, and after your workout, drink plenty of water and pick sports drinks without a lot of added sugar to replenish lost fluids and electrolytes.

Work out whenever it's convenient—just make sure that you don't eat a large or heavy meal within two hours of exercising. Don't train when you're hungry, either. Eat a protein or complex carbohydrate snack 30 to 45 minutes before your workout so you have some fuel for your body, or you may feel weak and shaky afterward. Good snacks include:

➠ Cheese slices

➠ Egg salad on whole-grain crackers

- Hardboiled eggs
- Health bars
- Nuts
- Peanut butter on banana or celery
- Smoothies
- Yogurt

After working out, remember to continue hydrating. Also, replenish fuel supplies with complex carbohydrates, and consume proteins to help with muscle building and repair.

Nutritional Supplements

Multivitamins. I recommend a good-quality multivitamin—pharmacy grade (USP) is the best, good manufacturing process (GMP) is acceptable—as insurance that you're getting all the nutrients you need for your health. This is especially important today, as the body may be more challenged by the production of less foods that are nutrient dense, and by an increase in environmental toxins.

Systemic enzymes. Not to be confused with digestive enzymes, systemic enzymes have long been touted in European studies as beneficial for a variety of general health reasons. Specifically, they're known to reduce the inflammation and muscle strain that often accompany intense exercise.

Other supplements. Digestive enzymes, probiotics, and omega fatty acids are other supplements that many of my patients take for general health.

Fitness Assessment

While it's certainly not necessary to do a fitness assessment before you begin an exercise program, I encourage you to do so for a couple of reasons. First, I think it's important to know what your baseline fitness level is (many people aren't even aware of what their resting pulse rate is) because it gives you important information about your health and connects you to your body. Second, if you're new to exercise and find it difficult in the beginning, having concrete, objective evidence of your physical fitness progress will serve to motivate you (although chances are, after a few sessions, you'll already look and feel better).

Heart rate. Knowing your resting heart rate gives you a snapshot of your overall heath. The average adult's resting heart rate is between 60 and 100, and usually will decrease as you become more fit. A lower heart rate means your heart doesn't have to work as hard, and studies on people with heart disease have shown that as heart rates climb up over 70 bpm, their risk of cardiovascular death increases.[28]

You can get your resting heart rate information from your family physician or a blood pressure monitor, or you can just take your pulse by placing the pads of your index and middle fingers on your opposite wrist, while the palm side of your wrist is face up, near the base of the thumb. Count the number of beats for 15 seconds and multiply that number by four to get your resting heart rate in beats per minute. You'll get the most accurate reading first thing in the morning, before getting out of bed.

Blood pressure. Your blood pressure is vital health information to know since high blood pressure leads to heart attacks and strokes, as well as other medical problems. You can contact your family physician for this information, or you can use a public or home blood pressure monitor.

Weight. Your weight is an easy thing to measure and a direct reflection of your fitness level. If you're overweight, you'll see your weight drop as you engage in HIIT. Since muscle weighs more than fat, however, weight alone is not always a good early measure of progress, as your muscle mass will increase as well. The way you look and feel will ultimately be the best reflection of your investment in this fitness program.

Height. Use the measure of your height in order to calculate your body mass index. And though some height loss is normal as we age, monitoring your height can also help alert you to the possibility of osteoporosis and compression fractures.

Body mass index. Calculating your body mass index (BMI) is useful to estimate body fat and gauge the risks associated with it. Higher BMIs put you more at risk for heart disease, type 2 diabetes, and certain cancers. You can plug in your height and weight into an online calculator to measure your BMI. The National Institutes of Health has one at https://www.nhlbi.nih.gov/health/educational/lose_wt/BMI/bmicalc.htm.

Cholesterol & fasting blood sugar. Cholesterol and fasting blood sugar information is important to know, as some of the most serious changes to your health first occur in these areas. This information should be available from your medical doctor, and is considered current if it's less than a year old. If any of these markers are abnormal, have them retested after you've been doing the HIIT exercises for a couple of months. You'll probably be impressed with the results and more motivated to make exercise a lifelong commitment.

Goal Setting

Goal setting can take you a long way toward achieving your desired level of health and fitness. There are a lot of different ways to set goals, but the two most important components are that your goals be written down, and that an action plan be incorporated. I recommend you buy yourself a notebook and document your journey. Here are the key elements of goal setting.

⇒ Write down your specific goals. For example: Lose 10 pounds, shed my belly fat, drop cholesterol 20 points, reduce blood pressure 10 points, get off diabetes medication.

⇒ Include your specific written plan. For example: Set the alarm clock for 7:00 a.m. tomorrow to exercise, purchase a yoga mat and sneakers, start stretching tonight after dinner.

⇒ Monitor your progress. Review your goals and plans weekly and determine if you met your goals or if they need to be adjusted.

⇒ Don't get discouraged. Habits take time to form; just keep at it if you fall short.

⇒ Reward yourself when you reach your goal. Buy those smaller pants, take a weekend trip, purchase a nice bottle of red wine.

In addition, or at a minimum if you're not a goal-setting person, I recommend that you write down the top five reasons you're embarking on this fitness path and what it is that you hope to gain from your efforts. Make your answers meaningful rather than just a list of items. In other words, instead of writing "to lose weight," write "to feel proud of myself and good about how I feel"; instead of "to live longer," write down "to be able to feel the joy of watching my youngest child get married"; instead of "to run a marathon," write down "to have the satisfaction of finally accomplishing one of my lifelong goals."

I also recommend you make a second list of the five most likely obstacles to your starting or sticking with an HIIT exercise program and, importantly, what emotional cost it will have if you allow those obstacles to stop you from acting. For me, an example of an obstacle would be finding the time and energy to exercise with two small children at home that I want to spend as much time with as possible. But the cost of not carving out a little time for HIIT (and, thankfully, it takes so little time) is not living as long or as healthily as I possibly could, and missing out on the joy of watching my daughters grow into adults.

Post these lists somewhere obvious (in sight = in mind) and read them every day. Use the power of your mind, and the motivating forces of pain and pleasure, to compel you into action. I guarantee it'll help you stay on track!

CHAPTER THREE

DYNAMIC WARM-UP

Proper warming up and cooling down are essential to getting the most out of your HIIT exercise routines—improving power and performance, as well as preventing injury. A popular way to warm up is to do dynamic stretches, which you should perform 5 to 10 minutes before your HIIT exercise. The foam roller exercises starting on page 112 are a great way to cool down the body and eliminate or reduce post-exercise muscle soreness. They can be done any time after, or between, workouts.

Dynamic warm-ups fall somewhere between static stretches and range-of-motion exercises. They move your body fluidly through a range of motion, and are held at the end points for a few seconds while the muscle stretches. They're important to use before your HIIT workout to warm up the muscles, loosen tendons and ligaments, and lubricate the joints. Though studies demonstrate that they can improve athletic performance, their primary role, as far as I'm concerned, is to prevent injuries.

To begin any dynamic warm-up, start in a balanced, neutral position, and deliberately and slowly follow the instructions for moving the target body part. Holding onto a counter or chair-back can make these maneuvers a little easier, help with balance, and prevent falls. Though very beneficial, dynamic stretches can irritate a tight and misaligned body if done too aggressively. Therefore, begin by doing just one or two reps of each exercise, and start with shorter ranges of movement. Increase the number of exercises and amount of movement after a week or two—each exercise should take only about 20 seconds total. While static stretches should be done daily, dynamic warm-ups should be done only two or three times a week, just before your HIIT workouts.

A couple of the dynamic warm-up exercises are the same or similar to HIIT exercises described later. Done slowly and deliberately, they can be an effective way to warm up the body. Done more rapidly—as during the HIIT workout—they serve to strengthen the body and get the heart rate pounding.

TRUNK SIDE BEND

1. Stand with your feet shoulder-width apart. Raise your left arm straight over your head and place your right hand on your hip. Bend your trunk laterally to the right as far as it will comfortably go.

2. Return to the center, switch arm positions, and then bend laterally to the left.

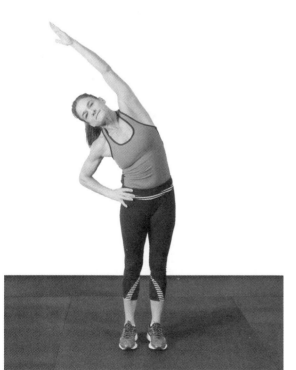

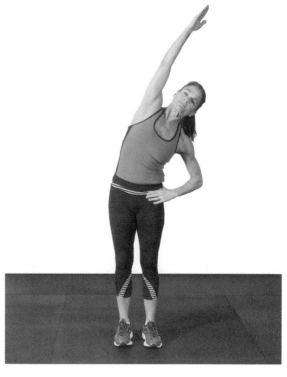

Return to starting position.

TRUNK ROTATION

1. Stand with your feet shoulder-width apart, arms out to the sides and parallel to the ground, elbows fully bent, and fists touching your chest. Rotate your upper body and head to the right as far as you can comfortably go so that you're looking over your right shoulder.

2. In a smooth motion, move back to the center and continue rotating to the left.

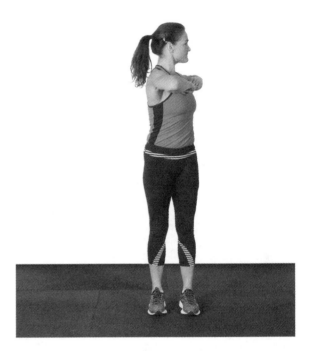

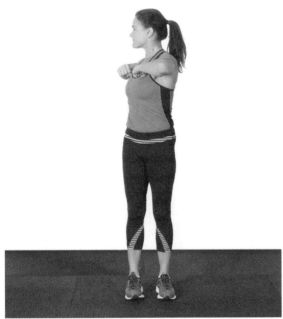

Return to starting position.

ARM CROSSOVER

1. Stand with your feet shoulder-width apart and arms extended straight out to the sides, level with your shoulders.

2. Simultaneously move your straight arms toward the center, crossing them in the middle of your chest, and continuing toward the other side.

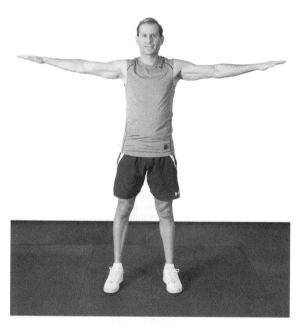

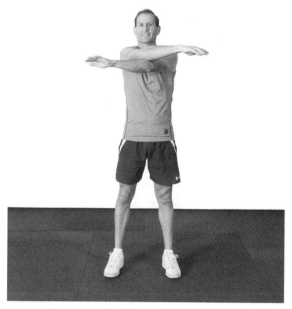

Move your arms back to the starting position and repeat, crossing the other arm on top.

ARM CIRCLE

1–2. Sit or stand with good posture. Bring both arms straight up and, in a continuous motion, bring them backward, down, then forward, forming a circle.

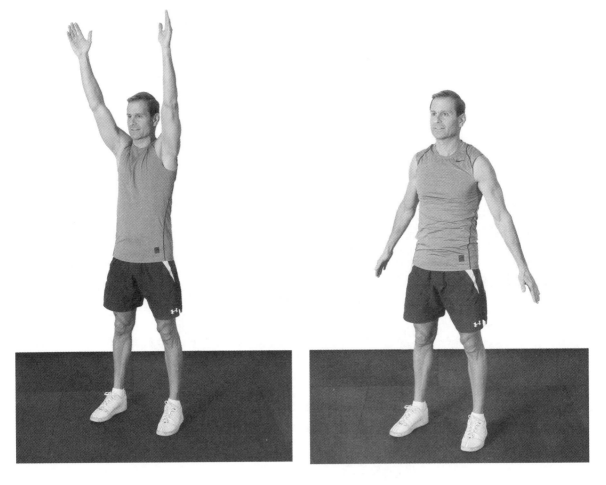

Repeat in the other direction.

SHOULDER BLADE MOBILITY

1. Start on all fours with your hands beneath your shoulders. Bring your right hand up and lightly place it on the back of your head with your elbow pointing to the side.

3. After a brief pause, move your elbow back up as far as you can comfortably go, rotating your head and shoulder with it, until your elbow is parallel to or above the floor, if possible.

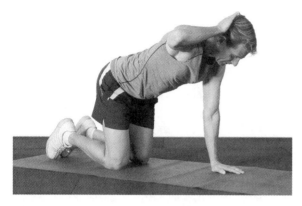

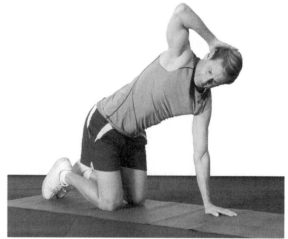

2. Now bring your right elbow down so that it points toward the floor, rotating your head and shoulder with it.

Switch sides and repeat.

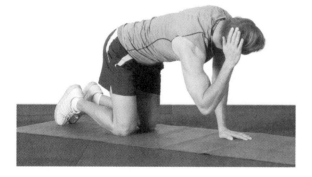

PAGE TURN

1. Lie on your right side with your knees pulled up and arms straight out in front of you.

2. Keeping your body in place, lift your left arm up and across your body toward the left side. Try to touch the ground on the left side.

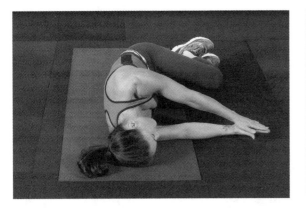

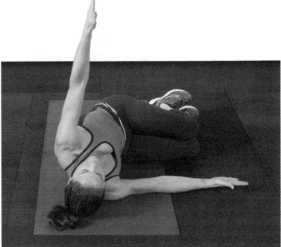

Return to starting position.

Switch sides.

Repeat several times.

SIDE LUNGE

1. Stand with your feet together and arms at your sides.

2. Take a large step to the right (wider than your shoulders), bending your right knee and shifting your weight and pelvis toward the right side. Keep your left leg straight as it drops toward the floor, coming up onto the right side of the left foot if needed. Maintain good upright posture of your trunk, and push your arms straight out in front of you for balance. Keep moving to the right side until you feel a stretch in the left groin area, at which point you should stop and return to the center.

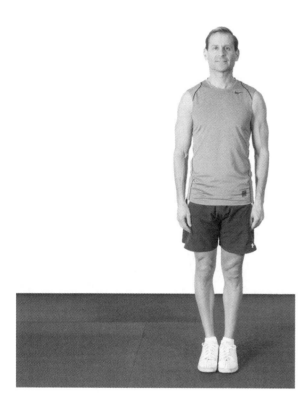

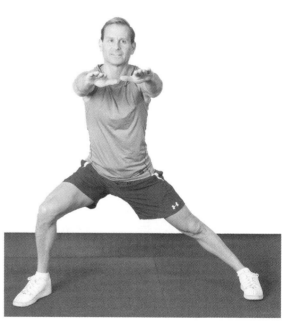

Switch sides and repeat.

KNEE TO CHEST

1. Stand with good posture and bring your right knee up toward your chest, grabbing your shin if you can as it comes close.

2. Let the right leg go and, as soon as it reaches the floor, bring the left knee up.

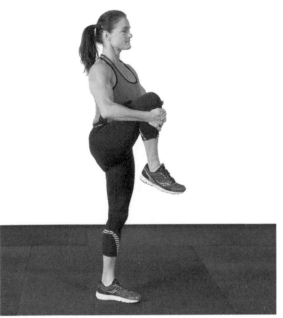

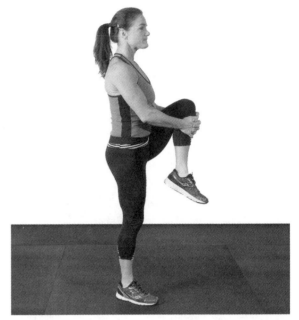

Let the left leg go and repeat.

Variation: Rising onto the toes of the leg on the floor may make it easier to grab the shin of the rising leg. Moving forward as you do this exercise may also make it easier.

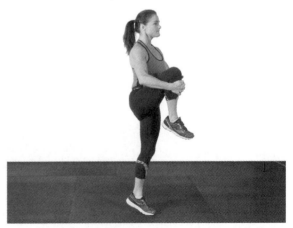

HIP STRETCH WITH A TWIST

1. Place your hands on the floor slightly in front of your shoulders, with arms and legs straight and your weight resting on the balls of your feet.

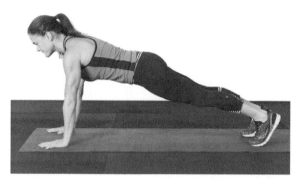

2. Keeping your back straight, bring your right foot close to your right hand. Try to keep your body from rising.

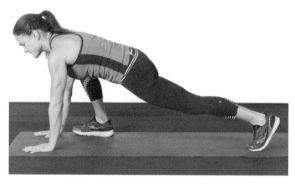

3. Lift your left hand off the floor and rotate your upper body as you extend your left arm and hand up toward the ceiling.

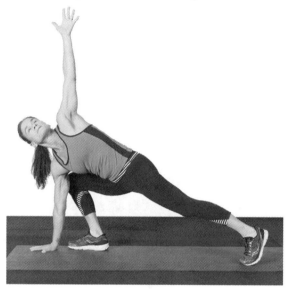

Lower your left arm and return to starting position.

Switch sides and repeat.

LEG CROSSOVER

1. Lie flat on your back with your legs straight and your arms extended out to the sides, forming a "T."

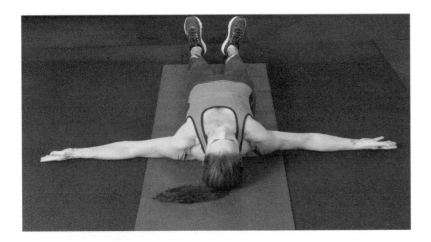

2. Bending your right knee, bring your right leg up and across your body, trying to touch your right foot to your left hand.

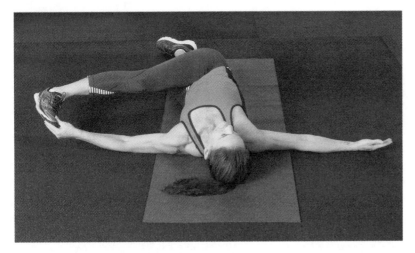

Return to starting position.

Switch sides and repeat.

HIP SWING

Go slowly with this exercise to avoid overworking the hip tendons and bursa.

1. Stand with your legs hip-width apart and hold onto a counter, wall, or other stable object for support. Keeping your right leg straight, slowly swing it forward to a comfortable height.

2. Keeping your upper body straight and abdominals slightly tightened, allow your leg to slowly come back down before swinging it behind you.

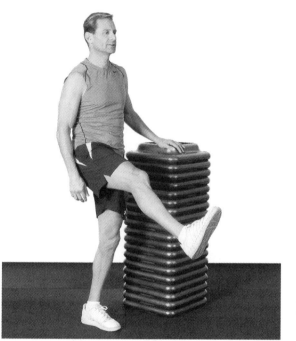

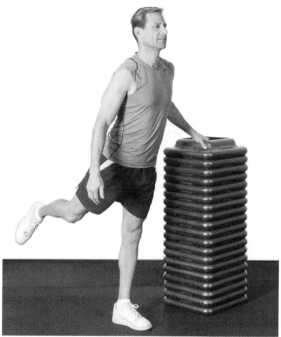

Repeat and then switch sides.

CHAPTER FOUR

HIIT ROUTINES

It took a little while to get here, but that's OK. Before starting with HIIT, it's important that you've adequately prepared by doing daily static stretches, occasional dynamic warm-ups, foam rolling, and moderate forms of aerobic conditioning.

Now that you've spent some time getting your body ready for this new challenge—you're probably already in the best shape you've been in years, you've documented your starting health status, and created your health and fitness goals—it's time to kick it into high gear! (*Note:* If you're the type to skip right to the exercises, don't. Go back and read Chapters Two and Three, especially the sections on avoiding injury!)

HIIT Strengthening

Chapter Five details over 40 different exercises that target the upper body, lower body, and core. There are beginner, intermediate, and advanced options for all fitness levels. While they can be used individually and mixed and matched in a variety of ways, I've created some HIIT routines to get you started. To give your body a complete workout, the routines include exercises from different categories, which also keeps the workout fun and interesting. There's also an additional workout routine specifically for improving posture, developed based on the information from my first book. Feel free to replace any of the exercises in the routines that irritate an existing area of pain, but avoid doing too many exercises in a row that target the same general muscles and body parts.

Many of the routines I've created take less than 10 minutes to complete (including warm-up time), which, based on the research of reduced-exertion high-intensity interval training (REHIIT), is enough to significantly improve your fitness level. Though the routines are short, you'll find that there's still plenty of room to progress and ratchet up the intensity of your workout.

As your fitness level improves, you'll naturally increase the number of repetitions of an exercise you can perform during the allotted time. You can also increase the workout interval lengths—e.g., do 30 seconds of intense exercise instead of 20—as well as the ratio of exercising time to resting time—e.g., instead of a 30-second workout followed by a 10-second rest (3:1), you can eliminate the rest period altogether (3:0).

If you're motivated to do even more, you can easily extend your workouts beyond the time allotted by adding another set or two of exercises at the end. While the science is still emerging, it appears that there are some additional benefits to longer interval workouts. Some REHIIT studies suggest that blood-sugar regulation and diabetes prevention may not be as effectively addressed with shorter-duration workouts, as compared to the more typical-length HIIT workouts.

Finally, I do not recommend using any additional weights—dumbbells, kettlebells, or medicine balls—until you've been doing the exercises for several weeks or more. Your own body weight will supply plenty of resistance to start. Once you can easily finish an exercise while maintaining good posture and form, you can incorporate some weights simply by holding them in your hands as you perform the exercise routines.

HIIT Cardio

The routines are the foundation of your HIIT fitness program. Done quickly and in succession, they will not only make you stronger, but also will give you a great cardio workout. However, if you enjoy walking, running, biking, swimming, or using cardio equipment like elliptical trainers, you can turn those activities into a HIIT session.

Once you've prepared your body for intense exercise and have properly warmed up, you can incorporate what the Swedes call *fartlek*, or speed-play, into your exercise routine. Perhaps you like to walk around a track or in the streets of your neighborhood. Next time you go out, try walking the track normally and then fast-walking or jogging the curves. Or choose two mailboxes or phone poles in the distance and pick up the pace as you move between them. If you're inside on an elliptical trainer or treadmill watching TV, try increasing your intensity during a commercial, and then go back to your regular pace when it's over.

If you're already fit and looking for a more high-powered workout, you could approximate one of the REHIIT workouts from a published study referred to earlier:

➡ Start your jog, bike, or swim with a 4-minute warm-up.

➡ Do a 10- to 20-second all-out sprint, pedal, or swim.

➠ Rest for 2 minutes.

➠ Sprint for another 10 to 20 seconds.

➠ Finish with a 3-minute cool-down.

As with the HIIT strength-training routines, you can easily increase the intensity of your cardio workout by increasing the exercise interval lengths or times, or by adding additional intervals. Here's a more intense format:

➠ Start your jog, bike, or swim with a 5-minute warm-up.

➠ Do a 10- to 20-second all-out sprint, pedal, or swim.

➠ Rest for 20 seconds.

➠ Do 5 to 8 sets of 10- to 20-second sprints followed by 20 seconds of rest.

➠ Finish with a 4-minute cool-down.

Putting It All Together

There are many ways to create a successful exercise routine for fitness and health. The only absolutes are that the routine includes both aerobic exercise and strength training, and that it be done regularly. While recommendations are constantly changing in the ever-evolving field of sports medicine—the new research on REHIIT hasn't even filtered down yet—most experts agree that 20 minutes or more of vigorous activity three days a week (more than that and you may be at greater risk for injury) plus at least two days a week of strength training is an effective overall fitness program.

To that end, I recommend that you start with one beginner workout from this book and, after a few weeks of training, add another HIIT routine per week from the book on a non-consecutive day. Eventually, the goal should be to perform two to three HIIT workouts per week, with at least two of them from this book—that would also fulfill your strength-training requirement. The third routine, if you decide to do one, can also be from this book, or you can add a day or two of moderate-pace activity such as a brisk walk or hike, or a different HIIT cardio routine like an interval swim in a pool.

Workout Gear & Equipment

One of the advantages of the HIIT workouts in this book is that you don't need any special equipment to do them. That makes HIIT an inexpensive and convenient method of exercise. Anywhere you can bring your body, you can use it to exercise.

There's some optional exercise gear, however, that you can use to enhance your workout, making it more comfortable and fun. Personally, I like to have gym and fitness "toys" lying around the house to remind and inspire me to get into action!

Footwear. Some of the exercises you can do barefoot, but others will be more comfortable with a lightweight supportive sneaker or exercise shoe.

Braces and supports. Many of my patients ask me if it's okay to wear knee braces, lumbar support belts, and other similar items while working out. I generally prefer that patients only wear support items when they must, like when doing heavy labor. However, if wearing a brace or support is the only way to comfortably exercise with a chronically painful joint or body part that has not responded to treatments or rest, then it's probably fine. Just be careful not to overwork a braced area.

Floor mat. With good sneakers, many of the HIIT exercises can be done on a hard floor. A carpeted space or floor mat will be more comfortable, however, for the exercises done down on the floor. I use an interlocking floor mat at home and a carpeted area at my office to do my workouts. Both work fine, as does a yoga mat, which is easy to travel with.

Step platform. Step-ups are included in the workout section because they're a great exercise for both cardio and leg strengthening. A staircase works great and is solid and cheap, but it only works if you have one handy. Otherwise, you can use a solid box, the seat of a sturdy park bench, or an adjustable step platform, which you can purchase at a retail or online sporting goods store.

Rebounder. Also known as a mini-trampoline, this is a popular apparatus for some of my patients. The benefits of bouncing up and down on this device are controversial. While experts argue the merits of it—how good an aerobic workout it provides, whether it provides lymphatic drainage, or if it helps with balance issues—one thing is certain: It's less taxing on your joints than many other forms of exercise. You can incorporate it into the routines if you find it easier on your body or more fun, but most of these exercises are low impact, and none require the use of a rebounder.

Watch/Timer. Timing your exercise intervals—both the high-intensity and the rest intervals—is important to keep you on track. You might find that even a 20-second high-intensity interval will go by faster when you're timing it. You may also find that you push yourself harder and get a better workout as you count it down. But remember: Never feel you must finish an exercise interval if you're feeling overworked or in pain.

Timing your intervals also serves to track your progress. The fitter you get, the more repetitions of an exercise you'll do within a set time interval, so be sure to count your reps as well. You may also decide at some point that it's time to increase the length of the high-intensity interval, shorten the rest interval, or both.

A watch with a second hand, a phone with a stopwatch or fitness app, or even a clock with a second hand are all acceptable methods to time the intervals.

Foam rollers. A whole new fitness niche has emerged around the use of foam rollers. In a nutshell, they're a great way to do some self-massage on sore and over-worked muscles. The result is often more relaxed muscles and other soft tissues, improved circulation, and less post-workout soreness. Information and specific exercises for foam rolling are covered in the Appendix.

Dumbbells, medicine balls, and kettlebells. The typical strength-training exercises that people associate with gyms, like using weight machines or free weights, are called isolation exercises because they usually work one or two specific muscles. The problem with isolation exercises is that they have the potential to build strength in an unbalanced way, thus creating injury and pain. The HIIT routines in this book, on the other hand, are called compound exercises because they engage multiple muscle groups and joints at the same time. Not only are compound exercises safer, they also have more practical, real-world applications.

The routines in this book primarily rely on your own body weight to supply the force. This is a very efficient way to work out, and makes it less likely for you to overdo it in the beginning. As you progress, however, you may want to incorporate the use of dumbbells, medicine balls, or kettlebells to keep challenging yourself to get stronger. Remember, if your muscles are strong enough to perform the task being asked of them, they won't devote extra resources toward getting stronger.

The amount of weight to use varies, but 3- to 5-pound dumbbells for women and 8- to 10-pound dumbbells for men is usually a good place to start.

Jump rope. Jumping rope can be a very fun way to get fit. If you decide to use a jump rope, here's how to size it: Place one foot in the center of the rope and lift the handles up. They should reach the level of your armpits.

Log book. A log book is a great tool for documenting your starting health statistics, your goals for exercise, and your progress as you go. You can monitor:

➡ The number of HIIT sessions per week

➡ The total time of the routine, and the individual workout and rest interval times

➡ The specific exercises done

➡ The number of repetitions of an exercise completed within the interval

Even starting out slowly, I think you'll be amazed at how quickly you progress.

The HIIT Routines

BEGINNER

This is where it begins. Incorporate these routines into your weekly exercise regimen, tailoring them to your fitness level, to begin your journey to ultimate health and fitness.

Note: Perform the dynamic warm-ups (page 32) for 4 minutes, then rest for 1 minute before beginning the routines.

ROUTINE 1

Total time: 5 minutes

Exercise 0:20 // Rest 0:10

1. Bird Dog (Legs Only), page 64

2. Knee Push-Up, page 81

3. Wall Slide, page 93

4. Jumping Rope, page 105

Rest 1 minute, then repeat the routine once.

ROUTINE 2

Total time: 5 minutes

Exercise 0:20 // Rest 0:10

1. Hip Raise, page 65

2. Triceps Dip, page 82

3. Knee-Down Lunge, page 94

4. Sprint, page 106

Rest 1 minute, then repeat the routine once.

ROUTINE 3

Total time: 5 minutes

Exercise 0:20 // Rest 0:10

1. Bent-Leg Kick Back, page 68

2. Floor Raise I-Y-T, page 84

3. Step-Up, page 95

4. Mountain Climber, page 107

Rest 1 minute, then repeat the routine once.

ROUTINE 4

Total time: 5 minutes

Exercise 0:20 // Rest 0:10

1. Turkish Get-Up, page 66

2. Jumping Jack Press, page 86

3. Sprint, page 106

4. Squat Thrust, page 108

Rest 1 minute, then repeat the routine once.

ROUTINE 5

Total time: 5 minutes

Exercise 0:20 // Rest 0:10

1. Hip Raise, page 65

2. Bent-Knee Side Plank, page 87

3. Mountain Climber, page 107

4. Ski Jump, page 110

Rest 1 minute, then repeat the routine once.

ROUTINE 6

Total time: 5 minutes

Exercise 0:20 // Rest 0:10

1. Bird Dog (Legs Only), page 64

2. Inchworm, page 88

3. Step-Up, page 95

4. Burpee (Optional Push-Up), page 111

Rest 1 minute, then repeat the routine once.

ROUTINE 7

Total time: 5 minutes

Exercise 0:20 // Rest 0:10

1. Bent-Leg Kick Back, page 68

2. Knee Push-Up, page 81

3. Knee-Down Lunge, page 94

4. Jumping Rope, page 105

Rest 1 minute, then repeat the routine once.

ROUTINE 8

Total time: 5 minutes

Exercise 0:20 // Rest 0:10

1. Turkish Get-Up, page 66

2. Jumping Jack Press, page 86

3. Mountain Climber, page 107

4. Burpee (Optional Push-Up), page 111

Rest 1 minute, then repeat the routine once.

ROUTINE 9

Total time: 5 minutes

Exercise 0:20 // Rest 0:10

1. Hip Raise, page 65

2. Inchworm, page 88

3. Step-Up, page 95

4. Ski Jump, page 110

Rest 1 minute, then repeat the routine once.

ROUTINE 10

Total time: 5 minutes

Exercise 0:20 // Rest 0:10

1. Bent-Leg Kick Back, page 68

2. Inchworm, page 88

3. Knee-Down Lunge, page 94

4. Jumping Jacks, page 104

Rest 1 minute, then repeat the routine once.

As you become more fit and find the above routines getting easier, you can move to the beginner plus routines. Or, you can continue with the beginner routines and lengthen the exercise intervals and/or adjust the ratio between the exercise and rest intervals.

For example, instead of Exercise 0:20 // Rest 0:10 (2:1), you could do Exercise 0:30 // Rest 0:10 (3:1) or Exercise 0:30 // Rest 0:00 (3:0).

BEGINNER PLUS

To increase your challenge even more, we've stacked two beginner routines on top of each other, increasing the challenge to your body and doubling the exercise time.

ROUTINE 1

Total time: 11 minutes

Exercise 0:20 // Rest 0:10

1. Bird Dog (Legs Only), page 64

2. Knee Push-Up, page 81

3. Wall Slide, page 93

4. Jumping Jacks, page 104

Rest 1 minute, then continue routine.

5. Hip Raise, page 65

6. Triceps Dip, page 82

7. Knee-Down Lunge, page 94

8. Sprint, page 106

Rest 1 minute, then repeat the whole routine from the top.

ROUTINE 2

Total time: 11 minutes

Exercise 0:20 // Rest 0:10

1. Bent-Leg Kick Back, page 68

2. Floor Raise I-Y-T, page 84

3. Step-Up, page 95

4. Mountain Climber, page 107

Rest 1 minute, then continue routine.

5. Turkish Get-Up, page 66

6. Jumping Jack Press, page 86

7. Sprint, page 106

8. Squat Thrust, page 108

Rest 1 minute, then repeat the whole routine from the top.

ROUTINE 3

Total time: 11 minutes

Exercise 0:20 // Rest 0:10

1. Hip Raise, page 65

2. Bent-Knee Side Plank, page 87

3. Mountain Climber, page 107

4. Ski Jump, page 110

Rest 1 minute, then continue routine.

5. Bird Dog (Legs Only), page 64

6. Inchworm, page 88

7. Step-Up, page 95

8. Burpee (Optional Push-Up), page 111

Rest 1 minute, then repeat the whole routine from the top.

ROUTINE 4

Total time: 11 minutes

Exercise 0:20 // Rest 0:10

1. Bent-Leg Kick Back, page 68

2. Knee Push-Up, page 81

3. Knee-Down Lunge, page 94

4. Squat Thrust, page 108

Rest 1 minute, then continue routine.

5. Turkish Get-Up, page 66

6. Jumping Rope, page 105

7. Mountain Climber, page 107

8. Burpee (Optional Push-Up), page 111

Rest 1 minute, then repeat the whole routine from the top.

ROUTINE 5

Total time: 11 minutes

Exercise 0:20 // Rest 0:10

1. Hip Raise, page 65

2. Inchworm, page 88

3. Step-Up, page 95

4. Ski Jump, page 110

Rest 1 minute, then continue routine.

5. Bent-Leg Kick Back, page 68

6. Inchworm, page 88

7. Knee-Down Lunge, page 94

8. Jumping Jacks, page 104

Rest 1 minute, then repeat the whole routine from the top.

ROUTINE 6

Total time: 11 minutes

Exercise 0:20 // Rest 0:10

1. Bird Dog (Legs Only), page 64

2. Knee Push-Up, page 81

3. Wall Slide, page 93

4. Jumping Rope, page 105

Rest 1 minute, then continue routine.

5. Turkish Get-Up, page 66

6. Jumping Jack Press, page 86

7. Sprint, page 106

8. Squat Thrust, page 108

Rest 1 minute, then repeat the whole routine from the top.

ROUTINE 7

Total time: 11 minutes

Exercise 0:20 // Rest 0:10

1. Hip Raise, page 65

2. Triceps Dip, page 82

3. Knee-Down Lunge, page 94

4. Sprint, page 106

Rest 1 minute, then continue routine.

5. Turkish Get-Up, page 66

6. Bent-Knee Side Plank, page 87

7. Mountain Climber, page 107

8. Ski Jump, page 110

Rest 1 minute, then repeat the whole routine from the top.

ROUTINE 8

Total time: 11 minutes

Exercise 0:20 // Rest 0:10

1. Bent-Leg Kick Back, page 68

2. Inchworm, page 88

3. Knee-Down Lunge, page 94

4. Jumping Jacks, page 104

Rest 1 minute, then continue routine.

5. Bird Dog (Legs Only), page 64

6. Knee Push-Up, page 81

7. Knee-Down Lunge, page 94

8. Squat Thrust, page 108

Rest 1 minute, then repeat the whole routine from the top.

ROUTINE 9

Total time: 11 minutes

Exercise 0:20 // Rest 0:10

1. Bird Dog (Legs Only), page 64

2. Knee Push-Up, page 81

3. Step-Up, page 95

4. Ski Jump, page 110

Rest 1 minute, then continue routine.

5. Hip Raise, page 65

6. Inchworm, page 88

7. Mountain Climber, page 107

8. Burpee (Optional Push-Up), page 111

Rest 1 minute, then repeat the whole routine from the top.

ROUTINE 10

Total time: 11 minutes

Exercise 0:20 // Rest 0:10

1. Bird Dog (Legs Only), page 64

2. Inchworm, page 88

3. Step-Up, page 95

4. Burpee (Optional Push-Up), page 111

Rest 1 minute, then continue routine.

5. Bent-Leg Kick Back, page 68

6. Floor Raise I-Y-T, page 84

7. Step-Up, page 95

8. Jumping Rope, page 105

Rest 1 minute, then repeat the whole routine from the top.

INTERMEDIATE

Here, we begin again with 5-minute routines. Don't be fooled, though; the exercises are decidedly more demanding, and the rests only come after completing the four exercises.

Note: Perform the dynamic warm-ups (page 32) for 4 minutes, then rest for 1 minute before beginning the routines.

ROUTINE 1

Total time: 5 minutes

Exercise 0:30 // Rest 0:00

1. Squat, page 96

2. Knee Push-Up with a Twist, page 89

3. Bird Dog, page 69

4. Jumping Jacks, page 104

Rest 1 minute, then repeat the routine once.

ROUTINE 2

Total time: 5 minutes

Exercise 0:30 // Rest 0:00

1. Lunge, page 97

2. Bear Crawl, page 90

3. Crunch, page 70

4. Sprint, page 106

Rest 1 minute, then repeat the routine once.

ROUTINE 3

Total time: 5 minutes

Exercise 0:30 // Rest 0:00

1. Reverse Lunge, page 98

2. Knee Push-Up with a Twist, page 89

3. Single-Leg Hip Raise, page 71

4. Mountain Climber, page 107

Rest 1 minute, then repeat the routine once.

ROUTINE 4

Total time: 5 minutes

Exercise 0:30 // Rest 0:00

1. Lateral Lunge, page 99

2. Bear Crawl, page 90

3. Plank, page 73

4. Ski Jump, page 110

Rest 1 minute, then repeat the routine once.

ROUTINE 5

Total time: 5 minutes

Exercise 0:30 // Rest 0:00

1. Lunge, page 97

2. Knee Push-Up with a Twist, page 89

3. Side Jackknife, page 72

4. Burpee (Optional Push-Up), page 111

Rest 1 minute, then repeat the routine once.

ROUTINE 6

Total time: 5 minutes

Exercise 0:30 // Rest 0:00

1. Squat, page 96

2. Bear Crawl, page 90

3. Single-Leg Hip Raise, page 71

4. Squat Thrust, page 108

Rest 1 minute, then repeat the routine once.

ROUTINE 7

Total time: 5 minutes

Exercise 0:30 // Rest 0:00

1. Reverse Lunge, page 98

2. Bear Crawl, page 90

3. Side Plank, page 74

4. Sprint, page 106

Rest 1 minute, then repeat the routine once.

ROUTINE 8

Total time: 5 minutes

Exercise 0:30 // Rest 0:00

1. Squat, page 96

2. Bear Crawl, page 90

3. Plank, page 73

4. Jumping Rope, page 105

Rest 1 minute, then repeat the routine once.

ROUTINE 9

Total time: 5 minutes

Exercise 0:30 // Rest 0:00

1. Lunge, page 97

2. Knee Push-Up with a Twist, page 89

3. Side Jackknife, page 72

4. Burpee (Optional Push-Up), page 111

Rest 1 minute, then repeat the routine once.

ROUTINE 10

Total time: 5 minutes

Exercise 0:30 // Rest 0:00

1. Lateral Lunge, page 99

2. Side Plank, page 74

3. Single-Leg Hip Raise, page 71

4. Ski Jump, page 110

Rest 1 minute, then repeat the routine once.

As you become more fit and find the above routines getting easier, you can move to the intermediate plus routines. Or you can continue with the intermediate routines and lengthen the exercise intervals and/or increase the ratio between the exercise and rest intervals.

For example, instead of Exercise 0:30 // Rest 0:00 (3:0), you could do Exercise 0:45 // Rest 0:10 (4.5:1).

INTERMEDIATE PLUS

To increase your challenge even more, we've stacked two intermediate routines on top of each other, increasing the challenge to your body and doubling the exercise time.

ROUTINE 1

Total time: about 11 minutes

Exercise 0:30 // Rest 0:00

1. Squat, page 96

2. Knee Push-Up with a Twist, page 89

3. Bird Dog, page 69

4. Jumping Jacks, page 104

Rest 1 minute, then continue routine.

5. Lunge, page 97

6. Bear Crawl, page 90

7. Crunch, page 70

8. Sprint, page 106

Rest 1 minute, then repeat the whole routine from the top.

ROUTINE 2

Total time: about 11 minutes

Exercise 0:30 // Rest 0:00

1. Reverse Lunge, page 98

2. Knee Push-Up with a Twist, page 89

3. Single-Leg Hip Raise, page 71

4. Jumping Rope, page 105

Rest 1 minute, then continue routine.

5. Lateral Lunge, page 99

6. Bear Crawl, page 90

7. Plank, page 73

8. Ski Jump, page 110

Rest 1 minute, then repeat the whole routine from the top.

ROUTINE 3

Total time: about 11 minutes

Exercise 0:30 // Rest 0:00

1. Lunge, page 97

2. Knee Push-Up with a Twist, page 89

3. Side Jackknife, page 72

4. Burpee (Optional Push-Up), page 111

Rest 1 minute, then continue routine.

5. Squat, page 96

6. Bear Crawl, page 90

7. Single-Leg Hip Raise, page 71

8. Squat Thrust, page 108

Rest 1 minute, then repeat the whole routine from the top.

ROUTINE 4

Total time: about 11 minutes

Exercise 0:30 // Rest 0:00

1. Squat, page 96

2. Knee Push-Up with a Twist, page 89

3. Bird Dog, page 69

4. Jumping Jacks, page 104

Rest 1 minute, then continue routine.

5. Reverse Lunge, page 98

6. Knee Push-Up with a Twist, page 89

7. Single-Leg Hip Raise, page 71

8. Mountain Climber, page 107

Rest 1 minute, then repeat the whole routine from the top.

ROUTINE 5

Total time: about 11 minutes

Exercise 0:30 // Rest 0:00

1. Lunge, page 97

2. Bear Crawl, page 90

3. Crunch, page 70

4. Sprint, page 106

Rest 1 minute, then continue routine.

5. Lateral Lunge, page 99

6. Bear Crawl, page 90

7. Plank, page 73

8. Ski Jump, page 110

Rest 1 minute, then repeat the whole routine from the top.

ROUTINE 6

Total time: about 11 minutes

Exercise 0:30 // Rest 0:00

1. Reverse Lunge, page 98

2. Knee Push-Up with a Twist, page 89

3. Single-Leg Hip Raise, page 71

4. Mountain Climber, page 107

Rest 1 minute, then continue routine.

5. Lunge, page 97

6. Knee Push-Up with a Twist, page 89

7. Side Jackknife, page 72

8. Burpee (Optional Push-Up), page 111

Rest 1 minute, then repeat the whole routine from the top.

ROUTINE 7

Total time: about 11 minutes

Exercise 0:30 // Rest 0:00

1. Squat, page 96

2. Bear Crawl, page 90

3. Single-Leg Hip Raise, page 71

4. Squat Thrust, page 108

Rest 1 minute, then continue routine.

5. Lunge, page 97

6. Bear Crawl, page 90

7. Crunch, page 70

8. Sprint, page 106

Rest 1 minute, then repeat the whole routine from the top.

ROUTINE 8

Total time: about 11 minutes

Exercise 0:30 // Rest 0:00

1. Lateral Lunge, page 99

2. Side Plank, page 74

3. Single-Leg Hip Raise, page 71

4. Jumping Rope, page 105

Rest 1 minute, then continue routine.

5. Reverse Lunge, page 98

6. Bear Crawl, page 90

7. Side Plank, page 74

8. Sprint, page 106

Rest 1 minute, then repeat the whole routine from the top.

ROUTINE 9

Total time: about 11 minutes

Exercise 0:30 // Rest 0:00

1. Lunge, page 97

2. Knee Push-Up with a Twist, page 89

3. Side Jackknife, page 72

4. Burpee (Optional Push-Up), page 111

Rest 1 minute, then continue routine.

5. Squat, page 96

6. Knee Push-Up with a Twist, page 89

7. Bird Dog, page 69

8. Jumping Jacks, page 104

Rest 1 minute, then repeat the whole routine from the top.

ROUTINE 10

Total time: about 11 minutes

Exercise 0:30 // Rest 0:00

1. Squat, page 96

2. Bear Crawl, page 90

3. Plank, page 73

4. Jumping Jacks, page 104

Rest 1 minute, then continue routine.

5. Lunge, page 97

6. Side Plank, page 74

7. Single-Leg Hip Raise, page 71

8. Squat Thrust, page 108

Rest 1 minute, then repeat the whole routine from the top.

ADVANCED

Here we begin again with 5-minute routines. Don't be fooled, though; the exercises are definitely even more demanding.

Note: Perform the dynamic warm-ups (page 32) for 4 minutes then rest for 1 minute before beginning the routines.

ROUTINE 1

Total time: 5 minutes

Exercise 0:30 // Rest 0:00

1. Prone Back Extension, page 75

2. Backward Bear Crawl, page 91

3. One-Leg Step-Up, page 100

4. Jumping Jacks, page 104

Rest 1 minute, then repeat the routine once.

ROUTINE 2

Total time: 5 minutes

Exercise 0:30 // Rest 0:00

1. Hip Up, page 76

2. Push-Up, page 92

3. Up & Down, page 101

4. Sprint, page 106

Rest 1 minute, then repeat the routine once.

ROUTINE 3

Total time: 5 minutes

Exercise 0:30 // Rest 0:00

1. Plank with Leg Raise, page 77

2. Backward Bear Crawl, page 91

3. Reverse Lunge with Reach, page 102

4. Mountain Climber, page 107

Rest 1 minute, then repeat the routine once.

ROUTINE 4

Total time: 5 minutes

Exercise 0:30 // Rest 0:00

1. Bicycle Crunch, page 78

2. Push-Up, page 92

3. Jumping Rope, page 105

4. Squat Thrust, page 108

Rest 1 minute, then repeat the routine once.

ROUTINE 5

Total time: 5 minutes

Exercise 0:30 // Rest 0:00

1. Lateral Bear Crawl, page 79

2. Backward Bear Crawl, page 91

3. One-Leg Step-Up, page 100

4. Ski Jump, page 110

Rest 1 minute, then repeat the routine once.

ROUTINE 6

Total time: 5 minutes

Exercise 0:30 // Rest 0:00

1. Circle Crunch, page 80

2. Push-Up, page 92

3. Up & Down, page 101

4. Burpee (Optional Push-Up), page 111

Rest 1 minute, then repeat the routine once.

ROUTINE 7

Total time: 5 minutes

Exercise 0:30 // Rest 0:00

1. Hip Up, page 76

2. Mountain Climber, page 107

3. Reverse Lunge with Reach, page 102

4. Jumping Jacks, page 104

Rest 1 minute, then repeat the routine once.

ROUTINE 8

Total time: 5 minutes

Exercise 0:30 // Rest 0:00

1. Plank with Leg Raise, page 77

2. Push-Up, page 92

3. Up & Down, page 101

4. Ski Jump, page 110

Rest 1 minute, then repeat the routine once.

ROUTINE 9

Total time: 5 minutes

Exercise 0:30 // Rest 0:00

1. Hip Up, page 76

2. Jumping Rope, page 105

3. Reverse Lunge with Reach, page 102

4. Burpee (Optional Push-Up), page 111

Rest 1 minute, then repeat the routine once.

ROUTINE 10

Total time: 5 minutes

Exercise 0:30 // Rest 0:00

1. Bicycle Crunch, page 78

2. Reverse Lunge with Reach, page 102

3. One-Leg Step-Up, page 100

4. Burpee (Optional Push-Up), page 111

Rest 1 minute, then repeat the routine once.

As you become more fit and find the above routines getting easier, you can move to the advanced plus routines. Or, you can continue with the advanced routines and lengthen the exercise intervals and/or increase the ratio between the exercise and rest intervals. For example, instead of Exercise 0:30 // Rest 0:00 (3:0), you could do Exercise 0:45 // Rest 0:10 (4.5:1) or Exercise 0:45 // Rest 0:00 (4.5:0).

ADVANCED PLUS

For the ultimate workout, we've increased your challenge even more. We've stacked two advanced routines on top of each other, as well as increased the exercise interval time and the total exercise time. Proceed with caution.

Note: Perform the dynamic warm-ups (page 32) for 4 minutes then rest for 1 minute before beginning the routines.

ROUTINE 1

Total time: About 18 minutes

Exercise 0:45 // Rest 0:10

1. Prone Back Extension, page 75

2. Backward Bear Crawl, page 91

3. One-Leg Step-Up, page 100

4. Jumping Jacks, page 104

Rest 1 minute, then continue routine.

5. Hip Up, page 76

6. Push-Up, page 92

7. Up & Down, page 101

8. Sprint, page 106

Rest 1 minute, then repeat the whole routine from the top.

ROUTINE 2

Total time: About 18 minutes

Exercise 0:45 // Rest 0:10

1. Plank with Leg Raise, page 77

2. Backward Bear Crawl, page 91

3. Reverse Lunge with Reach, page 102

4. Mountain Climber, page 107

Rest 1 minute, then continue routine.

5. Bicycle Crunch, page 78

6. Push-Up, page 92

7. Ski Jump, page 110

8. Squat Thrust, page 108

Rest 1 minute, then repeat the whole routine from the top.

ROUTINE 3

Total time: About 18 minutes

Exercise 0:45 // Rest 0:10

1. Lateral Bear Crawl, page 79

2. Backward Bear Crawl, page 91

3. One-Leg Step-Up, page 100

4. Ski Jump, page 110

Rest 1 minute, then continue routine.

5. Circle Crunch, page 80

6. Push-Up, page 92

7. Up & Down, page 101

8. Burpee (Optional Push-Up), page 111

Rest 1 minute, then repeat the whole routine from the top.

ROUTINE 4

Total time: About 18 minutes

Exercise 0:45 // Rest 0:10

1. Prone Back Extension, page 75

2. Backward Bear Crawl, page 91

3. One-Leg Step-Up, page 100

4. Jumping Jacks, page 104

Rest 1 minute, then continue routine.

5. Plank with Leg Raise, page 77

6. Backward Bear Crawl, page 91

7. Reverse Lunge with Reach, page 102

8. Mountain Climber, page 107

Rest 1 minute, then repeat the whole routine from the top.

ROUTINE 5

Total time: About 18 minutes

Exercise 0:45 // Rest 0:10

1. Hip Up, page 76

2. Push-Up, page 92

3. Up & Down, page 101

4. Sprint, page 106

Rest 1 minute, then continue routine.

5. Bicycle Crunch, page 78

6. Push-Up, page 92

7. Ski Jump, page 110

8. Squat Thrust, page 108

Rest 1 minute, then repeat the whole routine from the top.

ROUTINE 6

Total time: About 18 minutes

Exercise 0:45 // Rest 0:10

1. Plank with Leg Raise, page 77

2. Backward Bear Crawl, page 91

3. Reverse Lunge with Reach, page 102

4. Jumping Rope, page 105

Rest 1 minute, then continue routine.

5. Lateral Bear Crawl, page 79

6. Backward Bear Crawl, page 91

7. One-Leg Step-Up, page 100

8. Ski Jump, page 110

Rest 1 minute, then repeat the whole routine from the top.

ROUTINE 7

Total time: About 18 minutes

Exercise 0:45 // Rest 0:10

1. Circle Crunch, page 80

2. Push-Up, page 92

3. Up & Down, page 101

4. Burpee (Optional Push-Up), page 111

Rest 1 minute, then continue routine.

5. Hip Up, page 76

6. Mountain Climber, page 107

7. Reverse Lunge with Reach, page 102

8. Jumping Jacks, page 104

Rest 1 minute, then repeat the whole routine from the top.

ROUTINE 8

Total time: About 18 minutes

Exercise 0:45 // Rest 0:10

1. Hip Up, page 76

2. Mountain Climber, page 107

3. Reverse Lunge with Reach, page 102

4. Jumping Jacks, page 104

Rest 1 minute, then repeat the routine once.

5. Plank with Leg Raise, page 77

6. Push-Up, page 92

7. Up & Down, page 101

8. Ski Jump, page 110

Rest 1 minute, then repeat the whole routine from the top.

ROUTINE 9

Total time: About 18 minutes

Exercise 0:45 // Rest 0:10

1. Hip Up, page 76

2. Mountain Climber, page 107

3. Reverse Lunge with Reach, page 102

4. Burpee (Optional Push-Up), page 111

Rest 1 minute, then repeat the routine once.

5. Bicycle Crunch, page 78

6. Reverse Lunge with Reach, page 102

7. One-Leg Step-Up, page 100

8. Burpee (Optional Push-Up), page 111

Rest 1 minute, then repeat the whole routine from the top.

ROUTINE 10

Total time: About 18 minutes

Exercise 0:45 // Rest 0:10

1. Circle Crunch, page 80

2. Push-Up, page 92

3. Up & Down, page 101

4. Burpee (Optional Push-Up), page 111

Rest 1 minute, then continue routine.

5. Hip Up, page 76

6. Mountain Climber, page 107

7. Reverse Lunge with Reach, page 102

8. Burpee (Optional Push-Up), page 111

Rest 1 minute, then repeat the whole routine from the top.

Postural Improvement

Based on the information from my first book, the exercises in this routine are designed to combat years of harmful work and play habits. They strengthen the weak and compromised areas that commonly result from bad habits, which in turn reduces imbalance and improves posture. Performed once or twice a week, they can help to avoid injury and relieve pain.

Note: Perform the dynamic warm-ups (page 32) for 4 minutes then rest for 1 minute before beginning the routines.

Beginner: Exercise 0:20 // Rest 0:10 Total time: 6 minutes.

Advanced: Exercise 0:30 // Rest 0:00 Total time: 6 minutes.

1. Bird Dog, page 69

2. Shoulder Blade Squeeze, page 83

3. Wall Slide, page 93

4. Prone Back Extension, page 75

5. Floor Raise I-Y-T, page 84

Rest 1 minute, then repeat the whole routine from the top.

CHAPTER FIVE

THE HIIT EXERCISES

BIRD DOG (LEGS ONLY)

Level: Beginner

1. Start from your hands and knees in a flat-back (tabletop) position, with knees hip-width apart and hands shoulder-width apart.

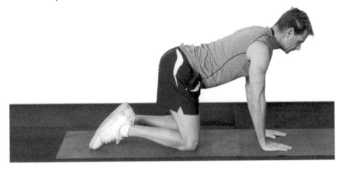

2. Engage your abdominal muscles by pulling your belly toward your spine. Keeping your neck and back in a straight line, lift your right leg and extend it straight back until it's parallel to the floor. Remember to keep looking straight down, and don't arch your lower back.

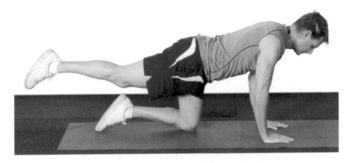

Hold for as long as you can maintain good form, up to half the allotted time interval.

Switch legs and repeat, holding for the other half of the allotted time interval.

HIP RAISE

Level: Beginner

1. Lie on your back with knees bent and feet flat on the floor. Place your arms out to the sides for stability.

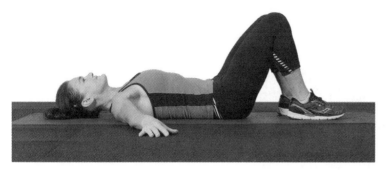

2. Clench your glutes and raise your hips up, forming a straight line from your thighs to your shoulders.

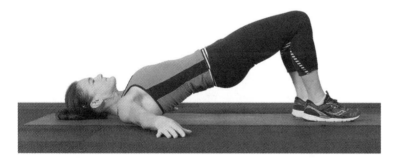

Keep your glutes engaged and hold the position at the top for a few seconds before lowering your hips back down to starting position.

Do as many repetitions as you can in the allotted time interval while maintaining good form.

TURKISH GET-UP

Level: Beginner

1. Lie on your back with legs extended, right arm at your side, and left arm pointing up to the ceiling.

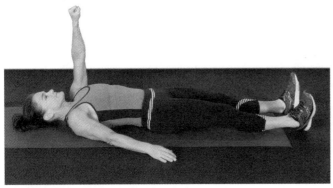

2–3. Keeping your left arm straight and pointing up, roll to your right side and use your right arm to assist you to a kneeling position.

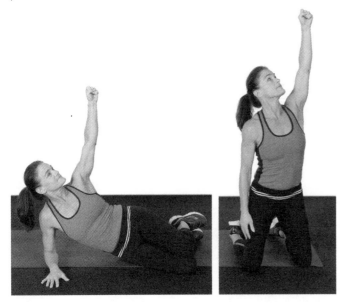

4. In a smooth motion, continue to a standing position.

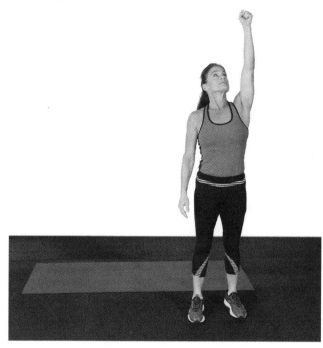

Reverse the movement to return to starting position, keeping the left arm elevated the whole time.

Switch arms and repeat.

Do as many repetitions as you can in the allotted time interval while maintaining good form.

BENT-LEG KICK BACK

Level: Beginner

1. Start on your hands and knees in a flat-back (tabletop) position, with knees hip-width apart and hands shoulder-width apart.

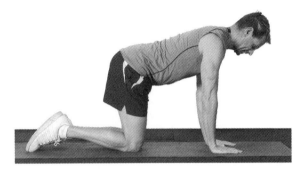

2. Engage your abdominal muscles by pulling your belly toward your spine. Keeping your right knee bent 90 degrees and your foot flexed, lift your right leg straight up behind you until your thigh is parallel to the ground and the bottom of your foot faces the ceiling.

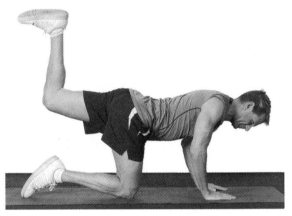

Hold for a couple of seconds and return to starting position.

Switch legs and repeat.

Do as many repetitions as you can in the allotted time interval while maintaining good form.

BIRD DOG

Level: Intermediate

1. Start from your hands and knees in a flat-back (tabletop) position, with your knees hip-width apart and hands shoulder-width apart.

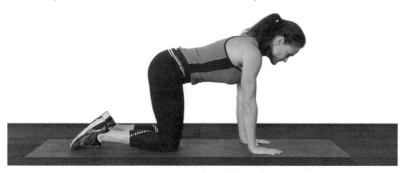

2. Engage your abdominal muscles by pulling your belly toward your spine. Look straight down and don't arch your lower back. While keeping your neck and back in a straight line, extend your left arm out in front of you at the same time as you extend your right leg behind. Both the leg and arm should be straight and parallel to the floor.

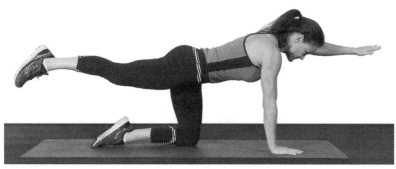

Hold for as long as you can maintain good form, up to half the allotted time interval.

Repeat with the other side and hold for the other half of the allotted time.

CRUNCH

Level: Intermediate

1. Lie on your back with knees bent and arms extended to the ceiling.

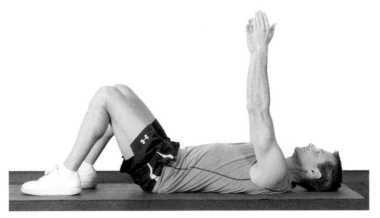

2. With your chin slightly tucked and abdominals tightened, curl up to bring your head and shoulders off the floor. Keep your neck relaxed and don't bring your head too far forward.

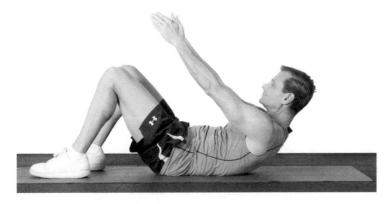

Slowly return to starting position.

Do as many repetitions as you can in the allotted time interval while maintaining good form.

SINGLE-LEG HIP RAISE

Level: Intermediate

1. Lie on your back with knees bent and feet flat on the floor. Place your arms out to the sides for stability. Raise your right leg and extend it at about a 45-degree angle.

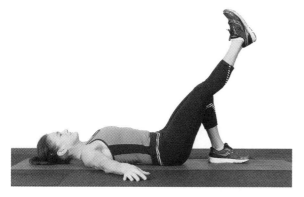

2. Raise your hips up, forming a straight line from your thighs to your shoulders. Clench your glutes as you rise and hold at the top.

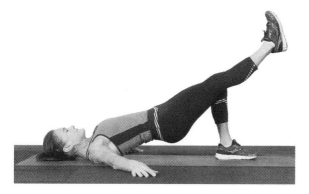

Pause a few seconds then lower your hips back down to starting position.

Switch legs and repeat on the other side.

Do as many repetitions as you can in the allotted time interval while maintaining good form.

SIDE JACKKNIFE

Level: Intermediate

1. Lie on your left side with your legs straight, right leg on top of the left. Place your right hand behind your head, with your elbow pointing toward the ceiling and your left arm extended on the floor in front of you for balance.

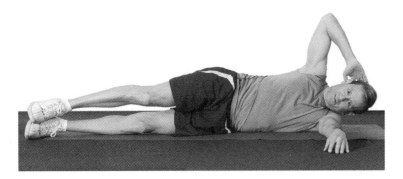

2. Engage your abdominals as you raise your right leg and simultaneously bend your upper body upward toward the raised leg, bringing your right knee and right elbow closer together.

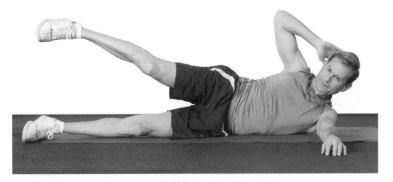

Do as many repetitions as you can in the allotted time interval while maintaining good form.

PLANK

Level: Intermediate

1. Lie facedown with your forearms underneath your chest and shoulders.

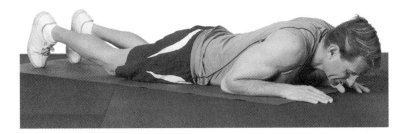

2. Prop yourself up on your forearms and come onto your toes. Your body should form a straight line from ankles to ears. Keep your head relaxed and facing the floor, and hold your core tight, pulling your belly toward your spine and keeping your butt muscles engaged. Hold for as long as you can maintain good form in the allotted time interval.

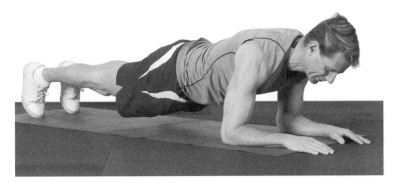

SIDE PLANK

Level: Intermediate

1. Lie on your right side with your right forearm and elbow resting on the floor in line with your shoulder. Keep your fingers pointed straight in front, your right hip on the floor, your left arm resting on your left hip, and your left leg stacked on your right leg.

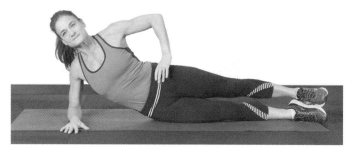

2. Tighten your core as you lift your hips off the floor until your body forms a straight line from feet to head. Keep your neck straight and relaxed with eyes looking forward. Continue holding your core tight by pulling your belly toward your spine and engaging your butt muscles. Hold for as long as you can maintain good form, up to half the allotted time interval.

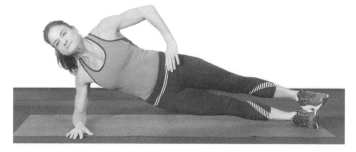

Repeat on the left side and hold for the other half of the allotted time.

PRONE BACK EXTENSION

Level: Advanced

1. Start on your belly with your elbows bent and hands slightly in front of your shoulders, legs straight, and feet resting on your toes. Keep your neck straight, looking down and slightly forward.

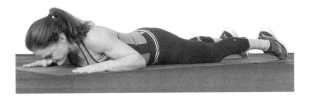

2. Keeping your arms and elbows tight against your sides, raise your hands a few inches off the floor.

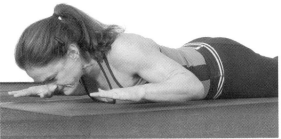

3–4. Lift just your chest up a few inches off the floor and then immediately lower it to starting position.

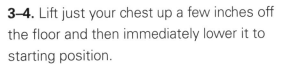

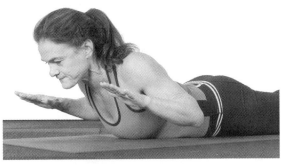

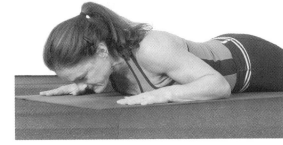

Do as many repetitions as you can in the allotted time interval while maintaining good form.

HIP UP

Level: Advanced

1. Lie on your right side with your right forearm and elbow resting on the floor in line with your shoulder. Keep your fingers pointed straight ahead, your right hip on the floor, your left leg stacked on your right leg, and your left arm resting on your left hip.

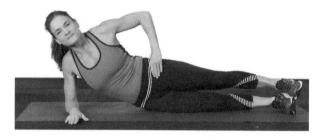

2. Tighten your core as you lift your hips off the floor until your body forms a straight line from feet to head. Keep your neck straight and relaxed with eyes looking forward.

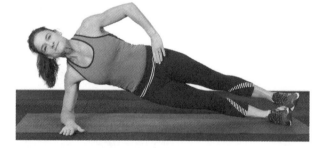

After a brief pause, drop your right hip back down to the floor to starting position.

Do as many repetitions as you can, maintaining good form, for up to half the allotted time interval.

Repeat on the left side and hold for the other half of the allotted time.

PLANK WITH LEG RAISE

Level: Advanced

1. Lie facedown on the floor with your forearms underneath your chest and shoulders. Prop yourself up on your forearms and come onto your toes. Your body should form a straight line from ankles to ears, with your head relaxed, looking down at the floor in front of you. Hold your core tight, pulling your belly toward your spine and engaging your butt muscles.

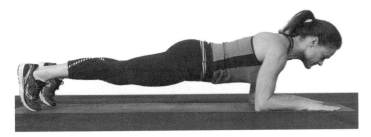

2. Lift your right leg 4 to 6 inches off the floor. Hold for as long as you can maintain good form, up to half the allotted time interval.

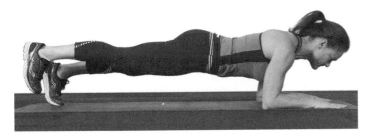

Repeat with the left leg, holding for up to the other half of the allotted time.

BICYCLE CRUNCH

Level: Advanced

1. Lie on your back with your hands behind your head and fingers interlocked. Engaging your abs, elevate your shoulders off the floor without pulling your head forward.

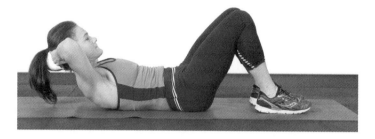

2. Lift both legs a few inches off the floor. Keeping your left leg steady, bring your right knee toward your chest and rotate your trunk by bringing your left arm and shoulder toward your bent knee. Hold the position briefly.

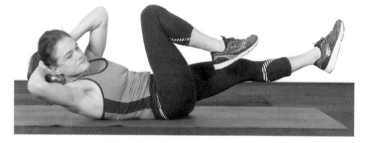

Switch sides and repeat.

Do as many repetitions as you can in the allotted time interval while maintaining good form.

LATERAL BEAR CRAWL

Level: Advanced

1. Start on all fours with your hands under your shoulders, knees bent under your hips, and heels off the ground. Raise your hips in the air while keeping a neutral spine. Keep your neck straight, eyes looking down and slightly forward.

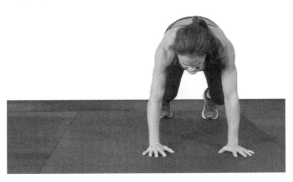

2. Starting with your left foot and right hand, crawl laterally to the right, using short movements. Don't rotate your body or cross your hands or feet as you move laterally.

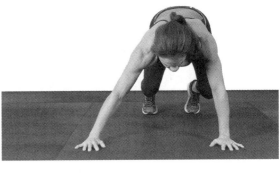

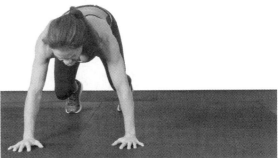

After several steps, crawl laterally to the left, starting with your right foot and left hand.

Do as many repetitions as you can in the allotted time interval while maintaining good form.

CIRCLE CRUNCH

Level: Advanced

1. Lie on your back with knees bent and feet flat on the floor. Place your hands behind your head, with elbows pointing to the sides.

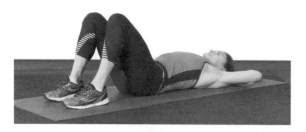

2. Lifting just the top of your back and shoulders up, engage your abdominals.

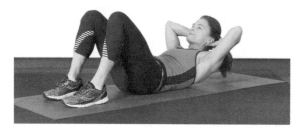

3–4. In one smooth motion, move your elevated upper body to the right by bringing your right elbow toward your right hip, roll toward the middle, and then finish by moving toward the left, bringing your left elbow toward your left hip.

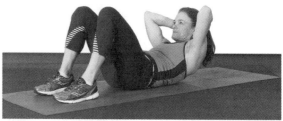

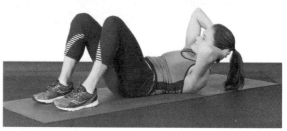

Lower the upper body to starting position. Repeat.

Do as many repetitions as you can in the allotted time interval while maintaining good form.

Upper Body

KNEE PUSH-UP

Level: Beginner

You can also use this exercise in your dynamic warm-up.

1. Place your hands on the floor slightly in front of your shoulders, with elbows bent 90 degrees and knees and toes on the ground. Keep your back and neck straight, while looking down and slightly forward.

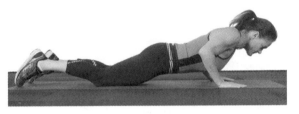

2. Raise your upper body with your arms, keeping your back straight and your knees and toes in contact with the floor the whole time.

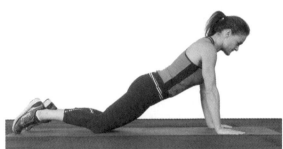

Once your arms are straight, lower yourself in a controlled manner back to the starting position.

Do as many repetitions as you can in the allotted time interval while maintaining good form.

TRICEPS DIP

Level: Beginner

1. Stand with your back to a chair seat or park bench. Bend your knees enough to reach behind you and place your palms on the seat. Keep your fingers facing forward and your arms straight.

2. Lower yourself by slowly bending your elbows to about 90 degrees, keeping them pointed straight back and your arms against your sides.

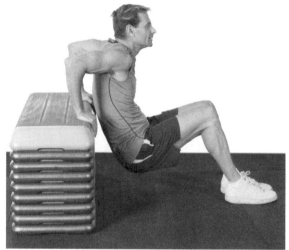

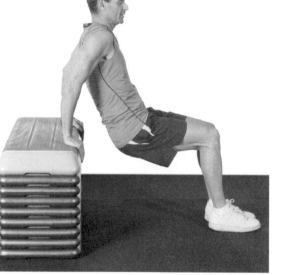

Push yourself up to starting position.

Do as many repetitions as you can in the allotted time interval while maintaining good form.

SHOULDER BLADE SQUEEZE

Level: Beginner

1. Lie on your back with your arms out to the sides and elbows bent 90 degrees. Your forearms should be perpendicular to the ground, with fists pointing up toward the ceiling.

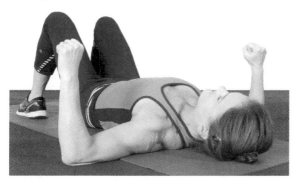

2. Push your elbows into the floor and squeeze your shoulder blades together toward you spine to lift your upper back slightly off the floor. Your pinching shoulder blades do the majority of work to lift you off the ground rather than your arms and shoulders.

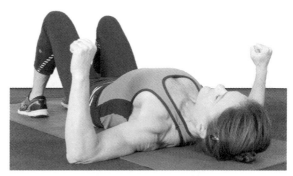

Hold for a few seconds before relaxing back to starting position.

Do as many as you can with good form in the allotted time interval.

FLOOR RAISE I-Y-T

Level: Beginner

These three positions target different parts of your upper back muscles. Choose one position per workout session, or alternate between two or three during a single session if you're fit enough.

I POSITION

1. Lie facedown with your arms extended over your head, forming a straight line, or letter "I." Keep your thumbs pointing straight up.

2. Slowly lift your arms up off the floor as far as you comfortably can.

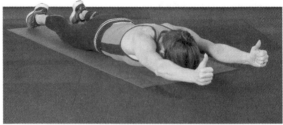

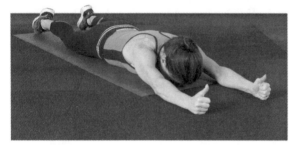

Lower them back to the starting position.

Do as many repetitions as you can in the allotted time interval while maintaining good form.

Y POSITION

1. Lie facedown with your arms extended out to the sides and angled in slightly toward your head.

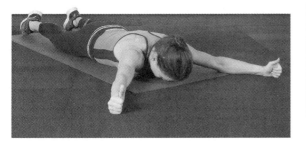

2. Slowly lift your arms up off the floor as far as you comfortably can.

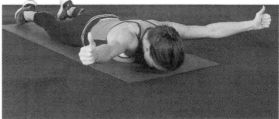

Lower them back to the starting position.

Do as many repetitions as you can in the allotted time interval while maintaining good form.

T POSITION

1. Lie facedown with your arms extended out to the sides.

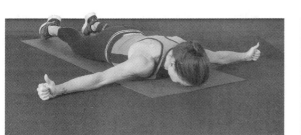

2. Slowly lift your arms up off the floor as far as you comfortably can.

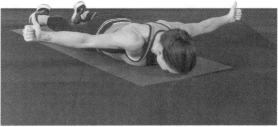

Lower them back to the starting position.

Do as many repetitions as you can in the allotted time interval while maintaining good form.

JUMPING JACK PRESS

Level: Beginner

1. Stand with your feet shoulder-width apart, arms at your sides.

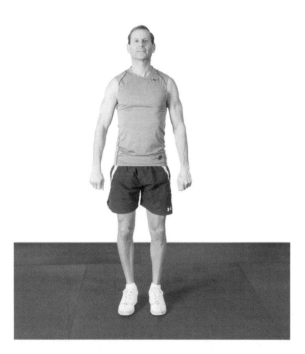

2. Begin by bending your elbows so that your fists are facing up. Jump your legs out wide while at the same time deliberately extending your fists straight up over your head.

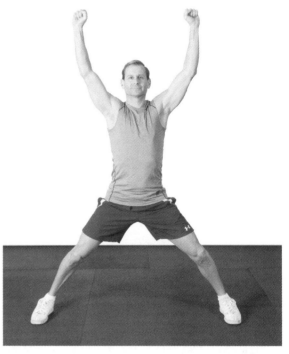

Jump your feet back together as you lower your arms back to your sides, keeping your elbows bent at your sides.

Do as many repetitions as you can in the allotted time interval while maintaining good form.

BENT-KNEE SIDE PLANK

Level: Beginner

1. Lie on your right side with your right forearm and elbow resting on the floor in line with your shoulder. Bend your knees 90 degrees and rest them on the floor, keeping your left leg on top of your right, with your left hand resting on your left hip.

2. Tighten your core as you lift your hips up to form a straight line from knees to head. Keep your core tight by pulling your belly toward your spine and engaging your butt muscles. Hold for as long as you can maintain good form, up to half the allotted time interval.

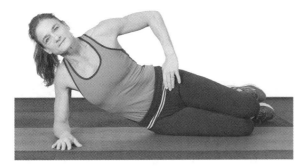

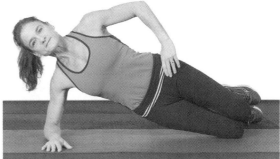

Repeat on the left side and hold for the other half of the allotted time.

INCHWORM

Level: Beginner

You can also use this exercise in your dynamic warm-up routine.

1. Start in a downward dog yoga pose, with your legs and arms straight and your hips high up in the air.

3. After a brief pause, walk your feet forward until they reach your hands, then slowly raise your body until you're standing tall.

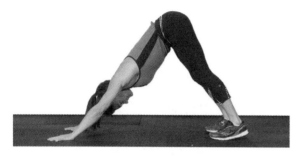

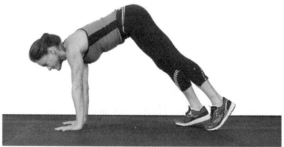

2. Keeping your legs and arms straight, walk your hands forward until your arms are under your shoulders and your body forms a straight line from head to toe (top position of a push-up).

4. Bending at the hips, not your lower back, reach your hands to the floor. Bend your knees if necessary.

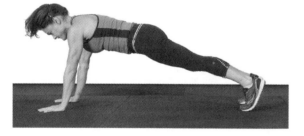

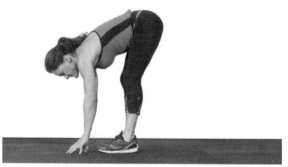

Walk your hands forward until you return to downward dog and repeat.

KNEE PUSH-UP WITH A TWIST

Level: Intermediate to Advanced

1. Place your hands on the floor slightly in front of your shoulders, with elbows bent 90 degrees and knees and toes on the ground. Keep your back and neck straight, while looking down and slightly forward.

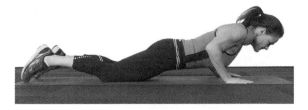

2. Keeping your knees and toes on the floor, lift your upper body with your arms.

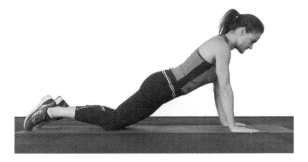

3. When your arms are straight, take your right hand off the floor and twist your body to the right to reach upward toward the ceiling.

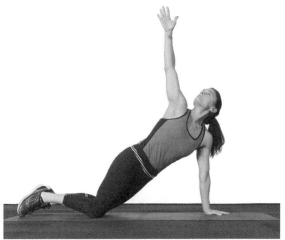

Drop your right arm back down and lower yourself in a controlled manner to starting position.

Repeat on the other side.

Do as many repetitions as you can in the allotted time interval while maintaining good form.

BEAR CRAWL

Level: Intermediate

This upper-body exercise also targets the core.

1. Start on all fours with your hands under your shoulders, knees bent under your hips, and heels off the ground. Raise your hips in the air while keeping a neutral spine. Keep your neck straight, eyes looking down and slightly forward.

2. With a relaxed, bear-like posture, crawl forward using short strides, starting with your right foot and left hand and following with your left foot and right hand.

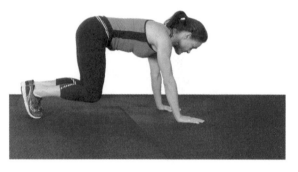

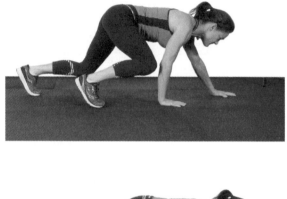

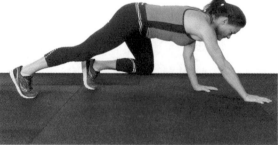

After several steps, turn and crawl back.

Do as many repetitions as you can in the allotted interval time while maintaining good form.

BACKWARD BEAR CRAWL

Level: Intermediate to Advanced

1. Start on all fours with your hands under your shoulders, knees bent under your hips, and heels off the ground. Raise your hips in the air while keeping a neutral spine. Keep your neck straight, eyes looking down and slightly forward.

2. Starting with your right foot and left hand, crawl backward using short strides and a relaxed posture.

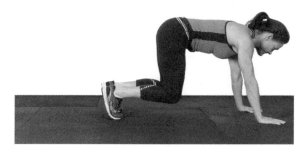

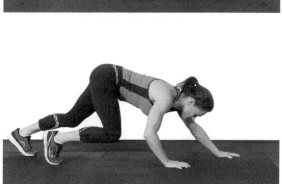

After several steps, turn around and walk backward in the other direction, or combine with the forward Bear Crawl (page 90).

Do as many repetitions as you can in the allotted time interval while maintaining good form.

PUSH-UP

Level: Intermediate to Advanced

1. Place your hands on the floor slightly in front of your shoulders with elbows bent 90 degrees and legs straight with your weight resting on your toes. Keep your back and neck straight with hips slightly up in the air while looking down and slightly forward.

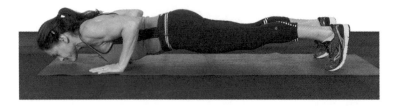

2. Raise your upper body with your arms, forming a straight line from toe to head. Hold your core tight, making sure your belly and butt muscles are engaged.

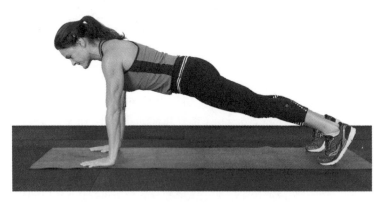

Once your arms are straight, lower yourself in a controlled manner until you reach the starting point.

Do as many repetitions as you can in the allotted time interval while maintaining good form.

Lower Body

WALL SLIDE

Level: Beginner

1. Start with your back against a wall, with your feet shoulder-width apart and a few feet from the wall. Look straight ahead and keep your head relaxed and shoulders back.

2. Slowly bend your knees and hips, pressing them slightly outward, and slide your upper back down the wall, feeling the resistance in your legs and butt muscles. Stop when your thighs are parallel or slightly below parallel to the floor. Your knees shouldn't extend past your toes.

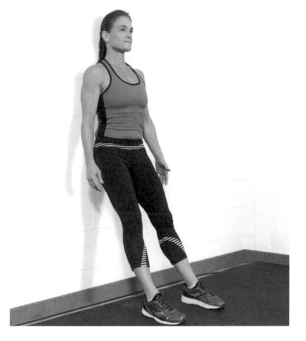

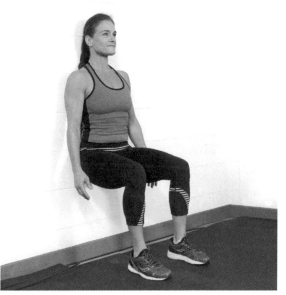

Slowly rise to starting position.

Do as many repetitions as you can in the allotted time interval while maintaining good form.

KNEE-DOWN LUNGE

Level: Beginner

1. Stand with your feet hip-width apart. Step your right foot forward and bend your knee 90 degrees so that your knee is perched above your ankle. Stay on the ball of your left foot and rest your left knee on a pad or mat directly under your left hip.

2. Keeping your upper body straight, press into your right foot and straighten your right leg. Hold this position.

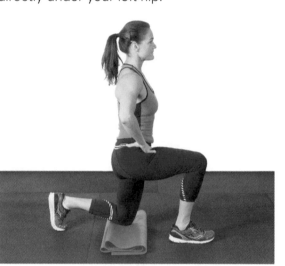

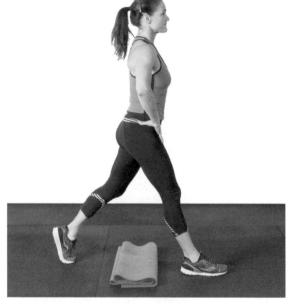

Return to starting position by bending your right knee and bringing your left knee back down to the mat.

Switch sides and repeat.

Do as many repetitions as you can in the allotted time interval while maintaining good form.

STEP-UP

Level: Beginner

1. Place your right foot on a sturdy step, bench, or chair.

2. Pressing your right heel into the step, bring your body up and land your left foot on the step next to your right foot.

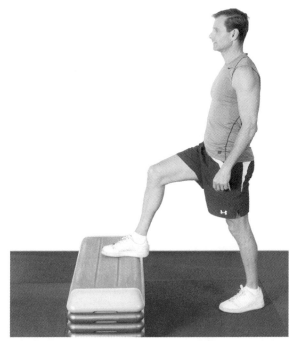

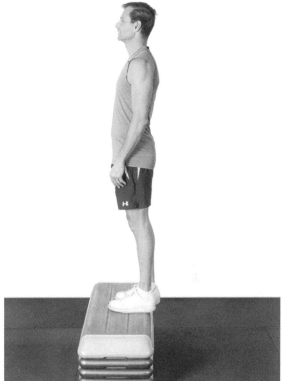

Bring your right foot back down to the floor, followed by the left. Repeat with the left leg leading.

Do as many repetitions as you can in the allotted time interval while maintaining good form.

SQUAT

Level: Intermediate to Advanced

Imagine you're standing on a towel and you're spreading it wider with your feet as you squat down. This will keep your knees from buckling inward.

1. Stand with feet slightly wider than shoulder-width apart, toes pointing slightly toward the sides.

2. Slowly bend your knees and hips, lowering your body as if you're going to sit down. Keep your torso straight, extending your arms out in front for balance. Keep your weight on your heels as you go into the squat, and don't let your knees extend past your toes. If possible, squat down far enough so that your thighs are parallel to the ground.

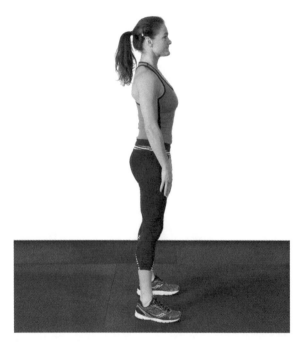

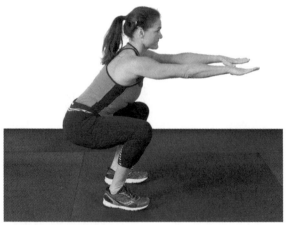

Return to starting position.

Do as many repetitions as you can in the allotted time interval while maintaining good form.

LUNGE

Level: Intermediate to Advanced

1. Stand with your feet shoulder-width apart and hands on your hips.

2. Take a big step forward with your right foot, bending your right knee to 90 degrees so that your right thigh is parallel to the floor. Your left thigh should be pointing straight down, with the knee hovering above the floor. Keep your upper body straight and don't let your front knee go pass 90 degrees.

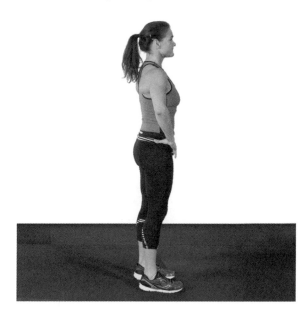

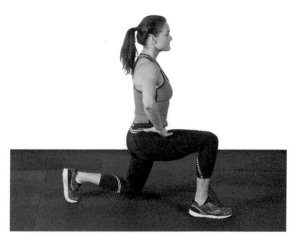

Step your right foot backward to return to standing position.

Switch sides and repeat.

Do as many repetitions as you can in the allotted time interval while maintaining good form.

REVERSE LUNGE

Level: Intermediate to Advanced

1. Stand with your feet shoulder-width apart and hands on your hips.

2. Take a big step backward with your right foot, bending the knee to 90 degrees so that the right thigh is pointing straight down with the knee hovering above the floor. The left thigh should be parallel to floor. Keep your upper body straight and don't let your front knee pass your ankle.

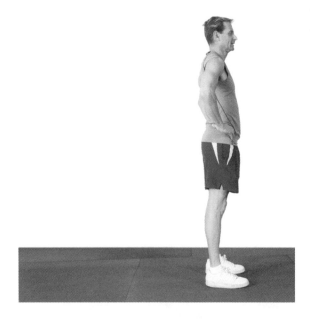

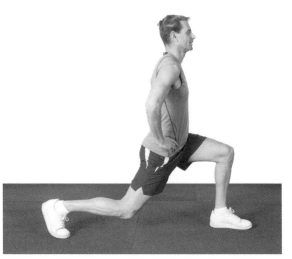

Step your right foot forward to return to standing position.

Switch sides and repeat.

Do as many repetitions as you can in the allotted time interval while maintaining good form.

LATERAL LUNGE

Level: Intermediate to Advanced

1. Stand with your feet shoulder-width apart and arms at your sides.

2. Step laterally to the left, keeping your weight on the heels and pushing your butt back, as if you were doing a squat. Keep your left knee in line with your left foot as you try to bring your left thigh parallel to floor.

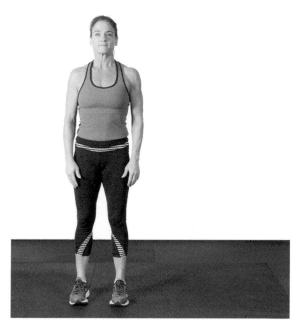

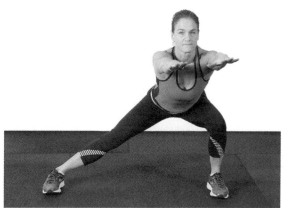

Push off your left leg to return to starting position.

Switch sides and repeat.

Do as many repetitions as you can in the allotted time interval while maintaining good form.

ONE-LEG STEP-UP

Level: Intermediate to Advanced

1. Place your right foot on a sturdy step, bench, or chair.

2. Pressing your right heel into the step, bring your body up, keeping the left knee bent and the left foot hovering above the ground. Hold the position briefly.

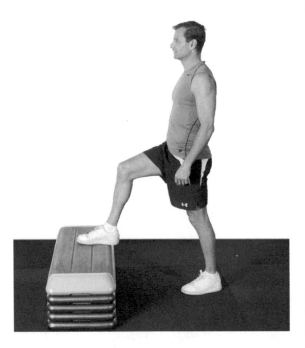

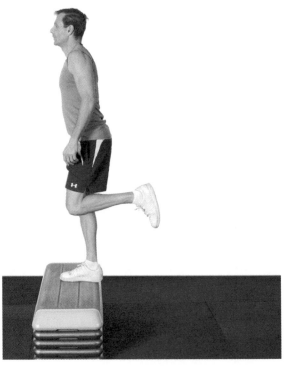

Return your left foot back to the floor, then bring your right foot back to the floor.

Repeat with your left foot leading the step up.

Do as many repetitions as you can in the allotted time interval while maintaining good form.

UP & DOWN

Level: Intermediate to Advanced

1. Start on your knees with good upright trunk posture.

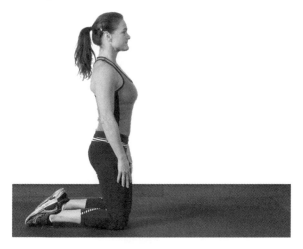

2. Bring your right leg forward so that your knee and hip are at 90 degrees. Keep your arms extended in front for balance.

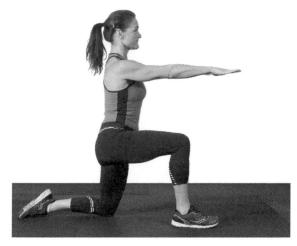

3. Bring your left leg forward so that your left foot lands next to your right. Your legs should now be shoulder-width apart in a squat position.

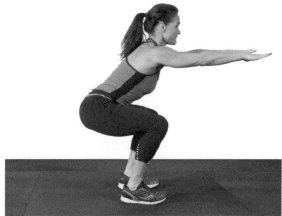

Bring your right foot back behind you into the kneeling position, followed by the left leg, returning you to starting position.

Repeat the exercise, alternating legs.

Do as many repetitions as you can in the allotted time interval while maintaining good form.

REVERSE LUNGE WITH REACH

Level: Intermediate to Advanced

You can also use this exercise in your dynamic warm-up routine.

1. Stand with your feet shoulder-width apart and hands on your hips.

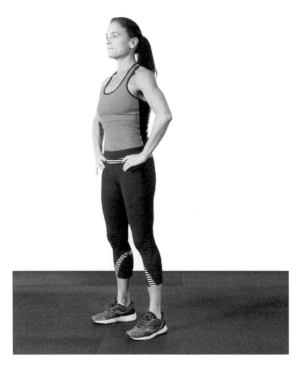

2. Take a big step backward with your right foot, bending your knee to 90 degrees so that your right thigh is pointing straight down, the knee hovering above the floor. Your left thigh should be parallel to floor. Keep your upper body straight and don't let your left knee pass your left ankle.

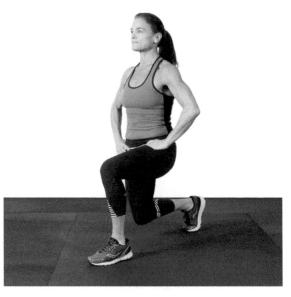

3. Reach your arms high overhead and tilt both arms over to your left side.

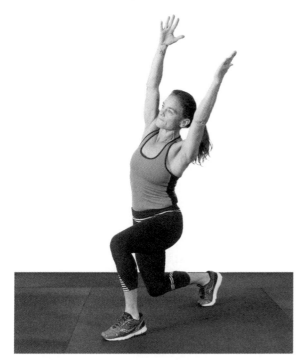

Step forward to return to starting position.

Switch sides and repeat.

Do as many repetitions as you can in the allotted time interval while maintaining good form.

JUMPING JACKS

Level: Beginner

1. Stand with your feet together and arms at your sides.

2. Jump your feet apart as you simultaneously swing your arms overhead. Land with your feet wider than hip-width apart.

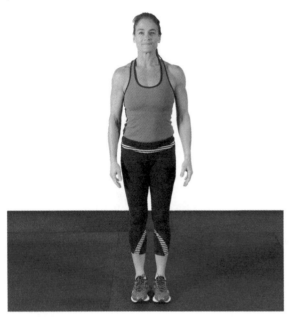

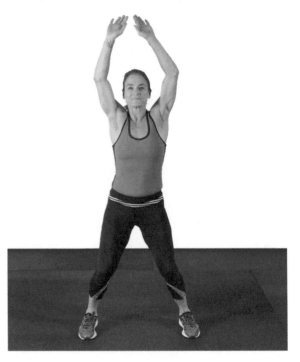

Jump your feet together and your arms back down to starting position.

Keep jumping as fast as you can in the allotted time interval while maintaining good form.

JUMPING ROPE

Level: Beginner

You can do these same motions without a jump rope.

1. Stand with your feet close together and arms at your sides. Hold one end of the jump rope in each hand, with the majority of the jump rope resting behind you on the floor.

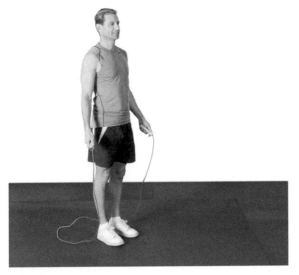

2–3. Maintain an upright posture as you swing the jump rope over your head and forward, jumping over it with both feet at the same time. Jump on the balls of your feet, lifting your heels off the ground and elevating your body 1 to 2 inches off the floor.

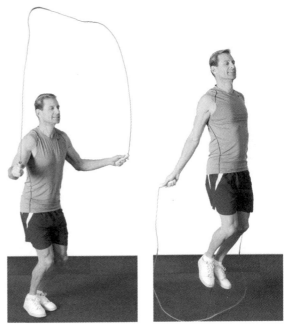

While swinging the rope, keep your hands at hip height with elbows slightly bent, and turn the rope using your wrists and forearms, keeping your shoulders relaxed and down.

Keep jumping as fast as you can in the allotted time interval while maintaining good form.

SPRINT

Level: Beginner

1. Stand with your feet hip-width apart.

2–3. Run or jog in place, bringing your knees up toward your chest. Keep your trunk upright with good posture. Pump your arms, with elbows bent, as if running, keeping your arm movements synchronized with your legs.

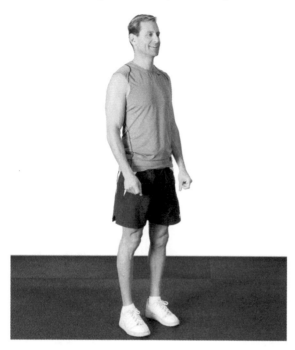

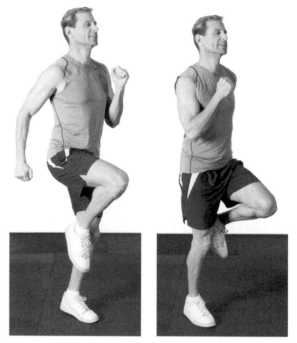

Continue for the allotted time interval while maintaining good form.

MOUNTAIN CLIMBER

Level: Beginner

This is also a great lower-body exercise.

1. Place your hands on the floor slightly in front of your shoulders with your arms straight, abdominals engaged, and body in a straight line from head to ankles. Keeping your back straight, bend your right knee and bring your leg up toward your chest.

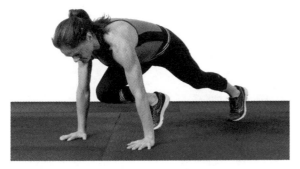

2. Quickly return your right leg to starting position and bend your left knee to bring your leg up toward your chest.

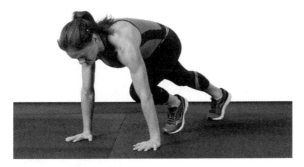

Alternate legs quickly while maintaining your posture.

Do as many repetitions as you can in the allotted time interval while maintaining good form.

SQUAT THRUST

Level: Intermediate

This is also a great core exercise.

1. Stand with your feet hip-width apart and arms hanging loosely. Bend your knees 90 degrees.

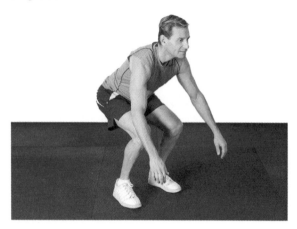

2–3. Reach down and place your hands flat on the floor in front of your feet, keep your arms straight, and thrust your legs back into the top position of a push-up. Keep your back straight, forming a straight line from your ankles to head.

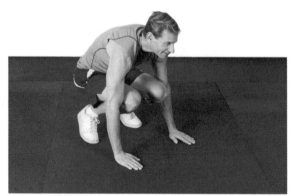

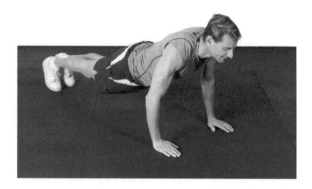

4. In a smooth motion, immediately jump forward to the starting position.

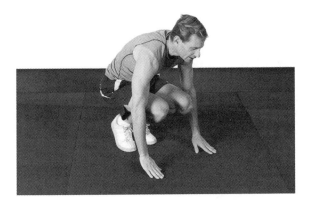

5. Keeping your core engaged, immediately stand up tall and extend your arms overhead.

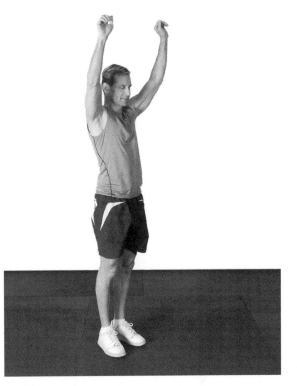

Return to starting position.

Do as many repetitions as you can in the allotted time interval while maintaining good form.

SKI JUMP

Level: Intermediate to Advanced

This is also a great lower-body exercise.

1. Stand with your feet together and bend your knees and hips slightly into a semi-squat position. Your weight should be on your heels and your trunk should be upright.

2–3. Keeping your feet close together and body facing forward, jump to the right, bringing your arms up in front of you for balance. Land softly in a half squat and immediately jump back to the left.

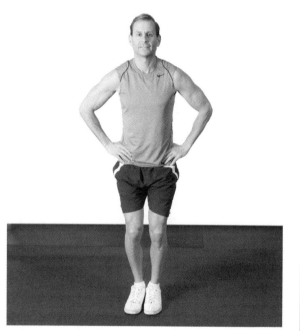

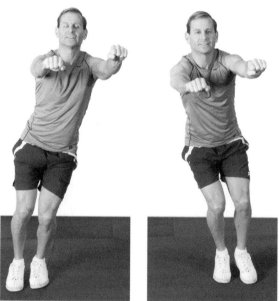

Alternate back and forth.

Do as many repetitions as you can in the allotted time interval while maintaining good form.

BURPEE (OPTIONAL PUSH-UP)

Level: Advanced

1. Crouch down with your feet shoulder-width apart and your hands on the floor near your feet, arms straight.

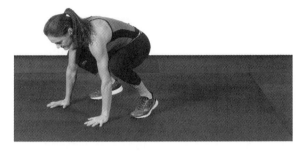

2. Jump both feet back into the top push-up position. Optionally, perform a push-up.

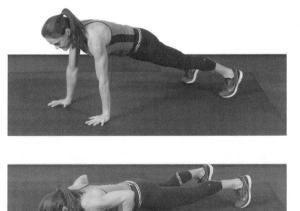

3. Jump your feet forward toward your hands back into a crouched position. Keep your weight on your heels.

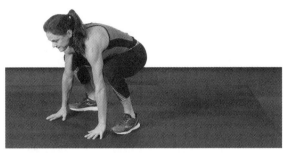

4. Immediately jump up with your arms outstretched overhead, making your body tall.

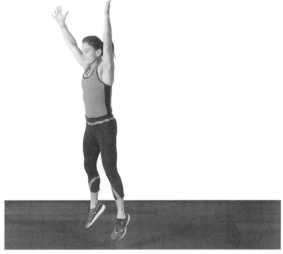

Land softly on the balls of your feet with your knees and hips flexed. Return to starting position.

Do as many repetitions as you can in the allotted time interval while maintaining good form.

APPENDIX

Foam Rolling

Self-massage techniques can relieve, as well as prevent, muscle and joint pain. I often recommend my patients use a foam roller to release tension, restore elasticity in the muscles and tendons, and promote circulation. It's been demonstrated that massage can reduce soreness and stiffness, and though I advocate professional bodywork, foam rollers are an inexpensive and convenient way to massage the muscles regularly.

I recommend a 6" x 18" or 36" round foam roller (the longer one makes it easier to roll both legs at once), which you can find online and at retail sporting goods stores. Don't buy a cheap one; they can be too soft and won't last. Look for a hard plastic tube covered in an inch or two of foam. Mine has grooves and spikes, designed for a better massage.

To use a foam roller, lie on a mat or carpeted surface and position the roller against the muscle, as described in the following pages. Let your body weight supply the force. Since you'll be using your arms on the floor for balance and support, you can also use them to control the amount of body weight and pressure being applied. Once in position, slowly roll back and forth over the muscle, moving the roller a few inches at a time. Spend a little more time on areas that are tender. Each muscle or area should take no longer than 30 seconds to complete. Roll along the muscles only, avoiding the joints.

Go slowly, and don't overdo it! Early on, while your muscles are still tight, some soreness afterwards is possible. That soreness is likely the result of the massage pressure breaking up restricted tissues and kicking up some inflammation in the process. Stop if it hurts, and try massaging that area again in a day or two, using less pressure. If you find that you're stopping a lot because of sore muscles, try using your foam roller on a bed to dial down the pressure even more.

I recommend using the foam roller regularly, and especially a few hours after your HIIT workout, to encourage circulation and reduce the post-workout soreness that sometimes occurs. A great time to foam-roll is while listening to music or watching TV.

GLUTES/PIRIFORMIS (BUTT MUSCLES)

1. Position the roller under your butt, leaning on one cheek. Place your hands on the floor behind you for support.

3. You can also turn your torso slightly from left to right to work the outer and inner sides of the butt muscles.

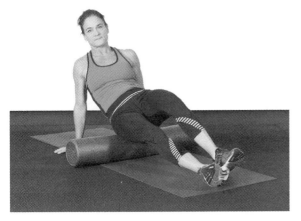

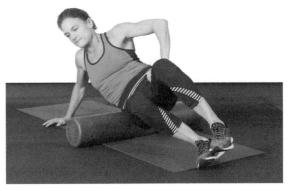

2. Move your body back and forth on the roller, from the top of your thigh to the base of your lower back.

Switch sides and repeat.

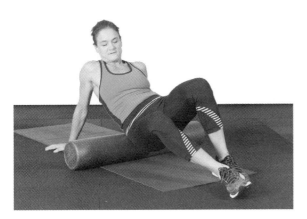

ILIOTIBIAL BAND

1. Place the roller on the side of your right thigh just below your hip, keeping your right forearm on the floor for support. Place your left foot flat on the floor in front of your right knee.

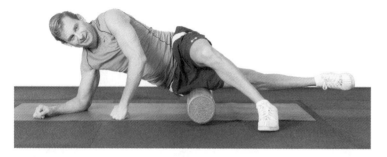

2. Move your body back and forth on the roller, a few inches at a time, from just below your hip to just above your knee.

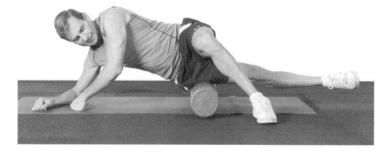

Switch sides and repeat.

GASTROCNEMIUS (CALVES)

1. Position the roller underneath your calves. Use your hands on the floor behind you for support, keeping your butt off the ground.

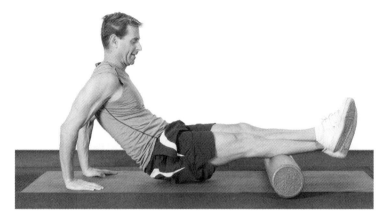

2. Move your body back and forth on the roller, from just below your knees to your ankles.

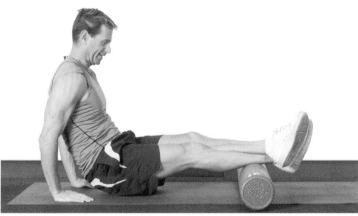

QUADRICEPS (FRONT OF THIGHS)

1. Lie facedown and place the roller under the fronts of both thighs. Place your forearms on the floor under your chest for support.

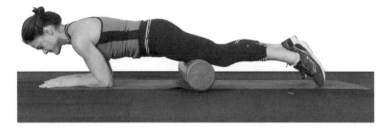

2. Move your body back and forth on the roller in small increments, from above your knees to the top of your thighs where they meet your pelvis.

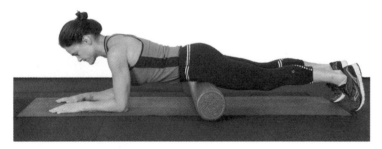

HAMSTRINGS (BACK OF THIGHS)

1. Sit on the floor and position the roller under both thighs with your legs extended forward. Place your arms behind you for support and elevate your butt off the floor.

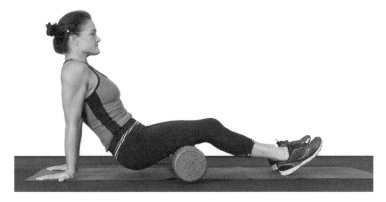

2. Move your body back and forth on the roller in small increments, from the base of your butt to just above the backs of your knees.

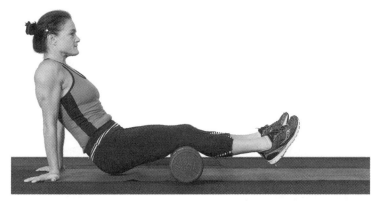

ERECTOR SPINAE (UPPER AND LOWER BACK)

1. Position the roller under your back, perpendicular to your spine, using your hands and body to support yourself as needed.

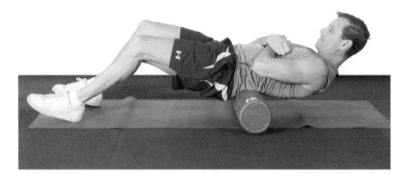

2. Move your body gently back and forth over the roller along the length of your spine, from your sacrum to the base of your neck. Avoid rolling your neck.

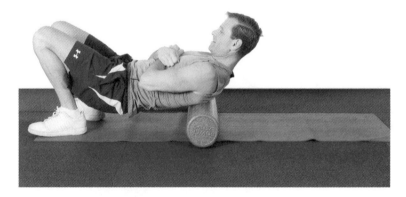

Static Stretches

Static stretches aren't generally recommended as a warm-up for exercise. However, when done regularly, they're a great vehicle for reducing tension in the muscles and other soft tissues, improving the alignment of the bones, and preparing the body for exercise. They're also easy to do, familiar to most everyone, and have been proven to be effective.

An example of a static stretch is when you bend at the waist and reach for your toes, holding the position steady for a certain number of seconds. In a static stretch, you remain still. Forget the bouncing and the pulling. Here are some other important points:

➡ *Hold the stretch* for approximately 30 seconds if you're younger than 65, and closer to 60 seconds if you're 65 or older. Holding a stretch for a shorter period has been shown to be less effective.

➡ *Do each stretch one time.* Though you may have to hold a stretch longer than you're used to, the good news is that doing several repetitions of each stretch, which a lot of people recommend, doesn't appear to improve the outcome significantly. "One and done," as they say.

➡ *Stretch every day.* Although there are studies that show results are possible from fewer days of stretching a week, doing them daily makes good sense. First, when you do something daily, it becomes automatic; you don't have to decide whether or not you can skip that day. And, second, the health of your musculoskeletal system is not static; you're either improving it or, by default, it's declining—we're getting tighter every day!

NECK STRETCH

Target: Cervical muscles

The back of your head should remain in contact with the floor, or pillow, at all times—you're sliding the back of your head along the floor, not lifting it up off the ground.

1. Lie on your back on the floor or in bed and let your head relax for a few seconds. Reach back and place the fingers of both hands in the space behind your neck, with your fingertips touching or fingers interlocked, and very gently move them up along the floor until they contact the back of your resting head. Keep moving your fingers up, pushing—or sliding—the back of your head up, feeling the back of the neck elongating. You may also notice that this movement tilts your head down and tucks your chin slightly.

Modification: If you have poor posture—especially if your head has moved significantly forward on your body—lying flat on your back on the floor or bed may be too uncomfortable. If that's the case, place as thin a pillow as you're comfortable with under your head. You can also put a pillow under your knees if your lower back is uncomfortable in this position.

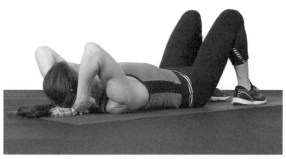

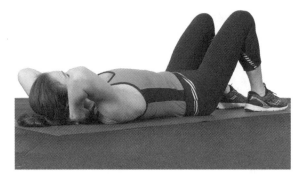

SHOULDER STRETCH

Target: Pectoralis muscles

1. Lie on your back with your knees bent and feet flat on the floor. Extend your arms out to the sides, palms up.

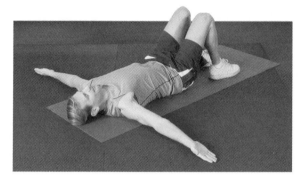

2. To stretch different parts of the chest and shoulder muscles, move your arms toward your head or hips, always keeping them on the floor.

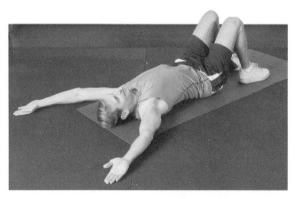

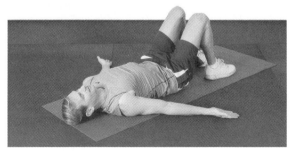

Intermediate Variation: If you don't feel a stretch in the shoulder or chest muscles when on the floor, try lying on a foam roller, foam bolster, or rolled-up towel along the length of your spine to increase the stretch. Your head should be supported by the roller itself or with a pillow of equal height.

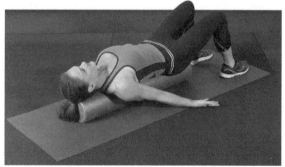

LOWER-BACK STRETCH

Target: Psoas muscles

The Position: Lie flat on your stomach with your forehead resting on the backs of your crossed hands. Relax your belly and feel the natural curve of your lower back. This may provide a sufficient stretch on its own.

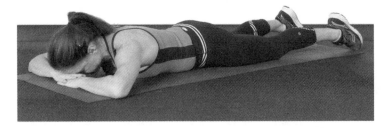

Variations: For more of a stretch, try coming up onto your elbows (the sphinx pose in yoga) or the palms of your hands (the cobra yoga pose). Remember, it's more important to relax the belly and let the lower back stretch gently than it is to try to go up higher.

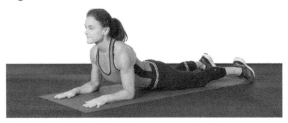

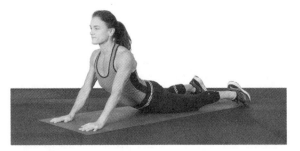

HIP STRETCH

Target: Piriformis muscles

1. Sit in a chair and rest your right ankle on top of your left thigh, just above the knee.

2. Gently hinge at the waist, leaning your upper body forward until you feel a stretch in your thigh/butt area. Make sure to keep your upper and lower back straight rather than letting them round. In other words, don't slump!

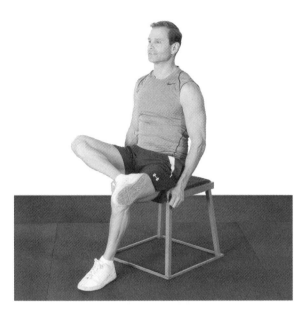

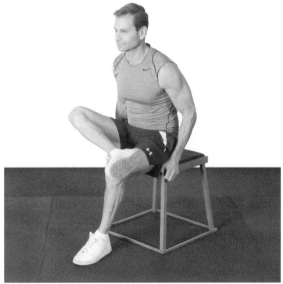

Switch sides and repeat.

BUTT STRETCH

Target: Gluteus muscles

1. Sit in a chair and rest your right ankle on top of your left thigh, just above the knee.

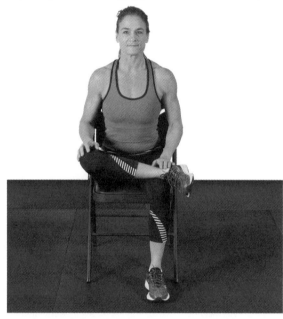

2. Grab your right knee with both hands. Leaving your right ankle resting on your left thigh, bring your right knee up and over across your stomach and toward your left side until you feel a stretch in the thigh/butt area. Think in terms of bringing your right knee as close to your left shoulder as possible, without lowering your shoulder or moving your right ankle from your left thigh.

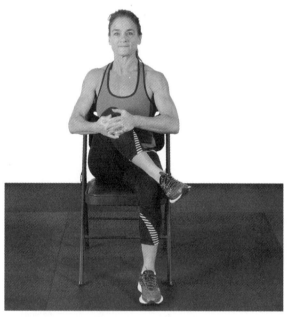

Switch sides and repeat.

FRONT OF THE THIGH STRETCH

Target: Quadriceps muscles

The Position: Stand with your left hand holding the back of a chair or other stable object for balance. Bend your right knee and grab your right ankle behind you with your right hand. Your right knee should be pointing down toward the floor. While holding the ankle in place, stand nice and tall, pushing your pelvis slightly forward. You should feel a gentle stretch in the front of your right thigh.

Variation: If you can't reach your ankle, loop a belt around it and grab that.

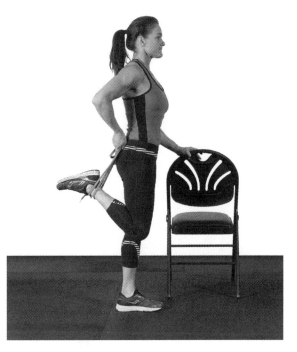

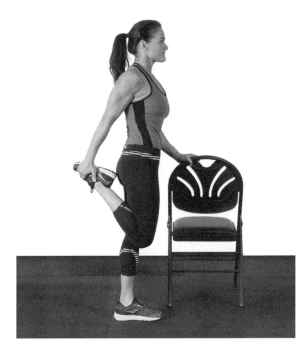

Switch sides and repeat.

BACK OF THE THIGH STRETCH

Target: Hamstring muscles

The Position: Stand with your right leg straight out in front of you with the heel resting on a chair seat, ottoman, or similar object, and bend forward at the hip joint. Don't slouch or round your back. You should feel a gentle stretch in the back of your right thigh.

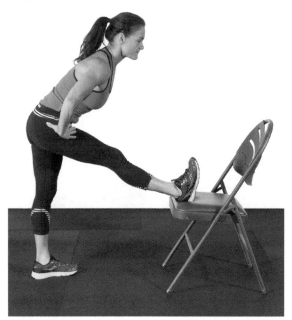

Switch sides and repeat.

CALF STRETCH

Target: Gastrocnemius muscles

The Position: Stand a few feet away from a chair, wall, or other stable object. Step forward with your right leg, bending at the knee, as you lean your body forward and hinge at the left ankle joint. Reach for the stable object with your outstretched arms. Make sure to keep your back straight as you lean forward and keep your left heel firmly planted on the ground. Move closer to or farther from the object until you feel a good stretch in the left calf muscle.

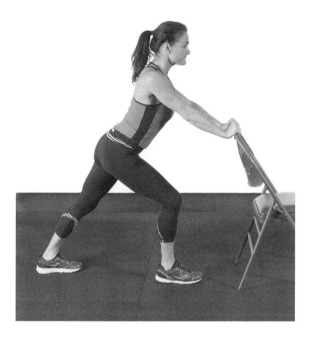

Switch sides and repeat.

SHIN STRETCH

Target: Anterior Tibialis muscles

1. Stand and hold onto a wall, chair, or counter for stability. Bend both knees slightly and place your right foot a few inches behind your left, with your right heel in the air and toes touching the ground (like a ballet dancer).

Switch sides and repeat.

Note: If you're flexible, this stretch can also be done while sitting on the floor, bending your legs underneath you, toes pointing behind you, with your butt sitting back on your heels. This stretches both shins at once.

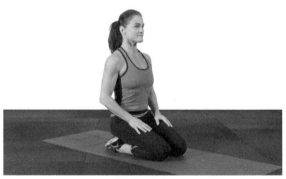

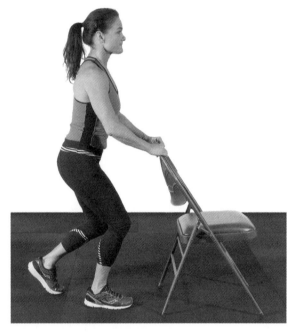

2. Pull your right leg forward without your right toes moving from their spot, causing your right heel to move forward, until a stretch is felt in the right shin.

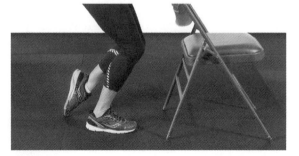

NOTES

1 Jacob S. Thum, Gregory Parsons, Taylor Whittle, and Todd A. Astorino. "High-Intensity Training Elicits Higher Enjoyment Than Moderate Intensity Continuous Exercise," *Plos One*, 12 (1) e0166299 (January 2017).

2 Amanda MacMillan. "Exercise Makes You Younger at the Cellular Level," *Time* (May 2017) http://time.com/4776345/exercise-aging-telomeres.

3 K. S. Weston, U. Wisloff, and J. S. Coombes. "High Intensity Interval Training in Patients with Lifestyle-Induced Cardiometabolic Disease: A Systematic Review and Meta-Analysis," *British Journal of Sports Medicine* 48 (16) (August 2014): 1227–1234.

4 J. S. Ruffino, P. Songsorn, M. Hagget, et al. "A Comparison of the Health Benefits of Reduced-Exertion High-Intensity Interval Training (REHIIT) and Moderate-Intensity Walking in Type 2 Diabetes Patients," *Applied Physiology, Nutrition, and Metabolism* 42 (2) (February 2017): 202–208.

5 L. J. Whyte, J. M. Gill, and A. J. Cathcart. "Effect of 2 Weeks of Sprint Interval Training on Health-Related Outcomes in Sedentary Overweight/Obese Men," *Metabolism*, 59 (10) (October 2010): 1421–8.

6 Matthew M. Robinson et al. "Enhanced Protein Translation Underlies Improved Metabolic and Physical Adaptations to Different Exercise Training Modes in Young and Old Humans," *Cell Metabolism*, Vol 25 (March 7, 2017): 581–592.

7 Ibid.

8 Gretchen Reynolds. "The Best Exercise for Aging Muscles," (March 2017) http://www.nytimes.com/2017/03/23/well/move/the-best-exercise-for-aging-muscles.html.

9 Zahra Mosallanezhad, Hojatollah Nikbakht, and Abbas Ali Gaeini. "The Effects of High-Intensity Interval Training on Telomerase Activity of Leukocytes in Sedentary Young Women," *International Journal of Analytical, Pharmaceutical and Biomedical Sciences*, Vol 3 (5) (November 2014): 39–43.

10 Gary O'Donovan, Andrew Owen, Steve R. Bird, et al. "Changes in Cardiorespiratory Fitness and Coronary Heart Disease Risk Factors Following 24 Wk of Moderate- or High-Intensity Exercise of Equal Energy Cost," *Journal of Applied Physiology* 98 (January 2005): 1619–1625.

11 R. B. Batacan Jr., M. J. Duncan, V. J. Dalbo, P. S. Tucker, and A. S. Fenning. "Effects of High-Intensity Interval Training on Cardiometabolic Health; A Systematic Review and Meta-Analysis of Intervention Studies," *British Journal of Sports Medicine* 51 (6) (March 2017): 494–503.

12 K. S. Weston, U. Wisloff, and J. S. Coombes. "High Intensity Interval Training in Patients with Lifestyle-Induced Cardiometabolic Disease: A Systematic Review and Meta-Analysis," *British Journal of Sports Medicine* 48 (16) (August 2014): 1227–1234.

13 O. Rognmo, T. Moholdt, H. Bakken, et al. "Cardiovascular Risk of High-Versus Moderate-Intensity Aerobic Exercise in Coronary Heart Disease Patients," *Circulation* 126 (12) (September 2012): 1436–1440.

14 Gary O'Donovan, Andrew Owen, Steve R. Bird, et al. "Changes in Cardiorespiratory Fitness and Coronary Heart Disease Risk Factors Following 24 Wk of Moderate- or High-Intensity Exercise of Equal Energy Cost," *Journal of Applied Physiology* 98 (January 2005): 1619–1625.

15 Alzheimer's Association. (October 23, 2017) www.alz.org.

16 Laura F. Defina, Benjamin L. Willis, et al. "The Association Between Midlife Cardiorespiratory Fitness Levels and Later-Life Dementia: A Cohort Study," *Annals of Internal Medicine* 158 (3) (February 2013): 162–168.

17 Stanley J. Colcombe, Kirk I. Erickson, et al. "Aerobic Exercise Training Increases Brain Volume in Aging Humans," *Journals of Gerontology. Series A. Biological Sciences and Medical Sciences* 61 (11) (November 2006): 1166–70.

18 Nicole Niemiec. "High Intensity Interval Training Reduces Stroke Risk 40 Percent," *Prevention* (February 2014). http://www.Prevention.com/print/health/health-concerns/hiit-reduces-stroke-risk-postmenopausal-women.

19 Joyce S. Ramos, Lance C. Dalleck, Arnt Erik Tjonna, Kassia S. Beetham, and Jeff S. Coombes. "The Impact of High-Intensity Interval Training Versus Moderate-Intensity Continuous Training on Vascular Function: A Systematic Review and Meta-Analysis," *Sports Medicine* 45 (5) (May 2015): 679–92.

20 Soren Moller Madsen, Anne Catherine Thorup, et al. "High Intensity Interval Training Improves Glycaemic Control and Pancreatic β Cell Function of Type 2 Diabetes patients," *Plos One* 10.1371 (August 2015).

21 R. B. Batacan Jr., M. J. Duncan, V. J. Dalbo, P.S. Tucker, and A. S. Fenning. "Effects of High-Intensity Interval Training on Cardiometabolic Health; A Systematic Review and Meta-Analysis of Intervention Studies," *British Journal of Sports Medicine* 51 (6) (March 2017): 494–503.

22   F. Maillard, S. Rousset, et al. "High-Intensity Interval Training Reduces Abdominal Fat Mass in Postmenopausal Women with Type 2 Diabetes," *Diabetes Metabolism* 42 (6) (December 2016): 433–441.

23   E. G. Trapp, D. J. Chisholm, J. Freund, and S. H. Boutcher. "The Effects of High-Intensity Intermittent Exercise Training on Fat Loss and Fasting Insulin Levels in Young Women," *International Journal of Obesity* 32 (4) (April 2008): 684–91.

24   M. Wewege, R. van den Berg, R. E. Ward, and A. Keech. "The Effects of High-Intensity Interval Training Vs. Moderate-Intensity Training on Body Composition in Overweight and Obese Adults: A Systematic Review and Meta-Analysis," *Obesity Reviews* 18 (6) (June 2017): 635–646.

25   Gary O'Donovan, Andrew Owen, Steve R. Bird, et al. "Changes in Cardiorespiratory Fitness and Coronary Heart Disease Risk Factors Following 24 Wk of Moderate- or High-Intensity Exercise of Equal Energy Cost," *Journal of Applied Physiology* 98, January 2005: 1619–1625.

26   R. B. Batacan Jr., M. J. Duncan, V. J. Dalbo, P. S. Tucker, and A. S. Fenning. "Effects of High-Intensity Interval Training on Cardiometabolic Health; A Systematic Review and Meta-Analysis of Intervention Studies," *British Journal of Sports Medicine* 51 (6) (March 2017): 494–503.

27   Chantal A. Vella, PhD and Len Kravitz, PhD. "Exercise Afterburn," https://www.unm.edu/~lkravitz/Article%20folder/epocarticle.html.

28   Kim Fox, Ian Ford, et al. "Heart Rate as a Prognostic Risk Factor in Patients with Coronary Artery Disease and Left-Ventricular Systolic Dysfunction (BEAUTIFUL): A Subgroup Analysis of a Randomized Controlled Trial," *Lancet* 372 (9641) (September 2008): 817–21.

BIBLIOGRAPHY

"2017 Alzheimer's Disease Facts and Figures." YouTube video, 1:45. Posted by actionalz (Alzheimer's Association) Mar 3, 2017. https://www.youtube.com/watch?time_continue=104&v=aLsVS0lrRD0.

Bartram, Sean. *High-Intensity Interval Training for Women: Burn More Fat in Less Time with HIIT Workouts You Can Do Anywhere*. New York: DK Publishing, 2015.

Bartman, Sean. *Idiot's Guide: High-Intensity Interval Training*. New York: Alpha Books/Penguin Random House, 2015.

Driver, James. *HIIT—High Intensity Interval Training Explained*. Lexington, KY: James Driver, 2012.

Hall, Roger. *Tabata Workout Handbook: Achieve Maximum Fitness with Over 100 High Intensity Interval Training Workout Plans*. Hobart, NY: Hatherleigh Press, 2015.

Mayo Clinic Staff. "Diabetes Complications." Mayo Clinic. July 31, 2014. Accessed August 15, 2017. http://www.mayoclinic.org/diseases-conditions/diabetes/basics/complications/con-20033091.

Metzl, Jordan D. *Dr. Jordan Metzl's Workout Prescription: 10, 20 & 30-Minute High-Intensity Interval Training Workouts For Every Fitness Level*. New York: Rodale Wellness, 2016.

Mosley, Michael, and Peta Bee. *Fast Exercise: The Simple Secret of High Intensity Training-Get Fitter, Stronger and Better Toned in Just a Few Minutes a Day*. New York: Atria, 2013.

Reynolds, Gretchen. "The Best Exercise for Aging Muscles." *New York Times*. Accessed August 15, 2017. https://www.nytimes.com/2017/03/23/well/move/the-best-exercise-for-aging-muscles.html.

Rooke, Kristin. "7 Interval Training Workouts to Burn Fat Fast." builtlean.com. Accessed August 15, 2017. Builtlean.com/2013/08/19/interval-training-workouts

Thapoung, Kenny. "You May Be Calculating Your Target Heart Rate Wrong." *Women's Health*. Accessed August 15, 2017. http://www.womenshealthmag.com/fitness/target-heart-rate.

Yeager, Selene. *The Women's Health Big Book of 15-Minute Workouts: A Leaner, Sexier, Healthier You—In 15 Minutes a Day!* New York: Rodale Inc., 2011.

INDEX

ACKNOWLEDGMENTS

A heartfelt thanks to Casie Vogel, Claire Chun, Shayna Keyles, Lily Chou, and the rest of the team at Ulysses Press for putting their faith in me to write another book, and then for making it better!

To two real American heroes, Dr. Andrew Taylor Still and Dr. William Garner Sutherland, for leaving a legacy of healing that I was fortunate to follow. And to the thousands of patients, and readers, who put their faith in my experience and knowledge—thank you.

And of course, a special thanks to my family. My darling wife, Janice, a true partner in love and life, and a wonderful mother to our children: You make it all possible, and fun! To my sweet little Lexi: Thank you for sacrificing some "daddy time" so that I could write. I miss every moment I'm not playing with you. And to littlest Madie, a ray of sunshine, here's to having another book of daddy's in the house for you to chew on. Finally, to my Mom: We're so happy to have you, grandma, as our new neighbor.

ABOUT THE AUTHOR

Dr. Joseph Tieri is an osteopathic physician and a specialist in the holistic, hands-on healing practice, of osteopathic manipulation. He is part owner and partner of the Stone Ridge Healing Arts Center, and has been in private practice for more than 17 years.

Dr. Tieri is the author of *End Everyday Pain for 50+: A 10-Minute-a-Day Program of Stretching, Strengthening, and Movement to Break the Grip of Pain*, and has published articles and editorials on osteopathy and holistic healing in the regional press and in the *Journal of the American Osteopathic Association*. He is an adjunct professor at Touro College of Osteopathic Medicine and a clinical instructor, teaching the art of hands-on osteopathy to medical students and residents in his office.

For more information, please visit endeverydaypain.com.